P9-CQC-350

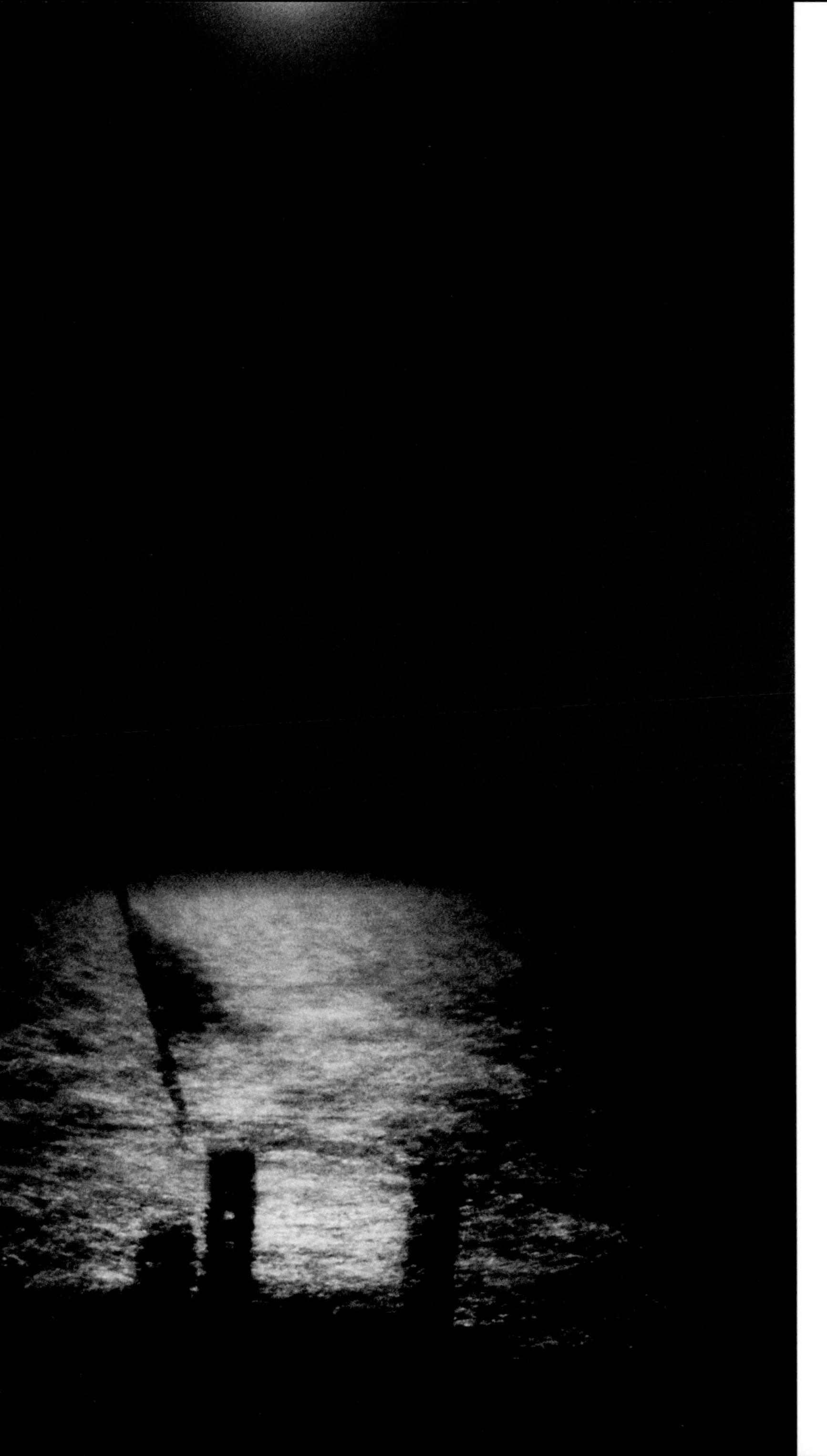

IMPRESSIONS

A gathering of poems and images,
neither conceived with knowledge of the other.

to and for my wife, Jan, and
our daughters, Jenny and Katie,
with gratitude for their infinite
patience, thoughtful insight and
discerning encouragement.

john erickson

Flowers at Prince Eugen's Home, Stockholm, Sweden 1997

Evening, Carmel Beach, Carmel-by-the-Sea, California 2001

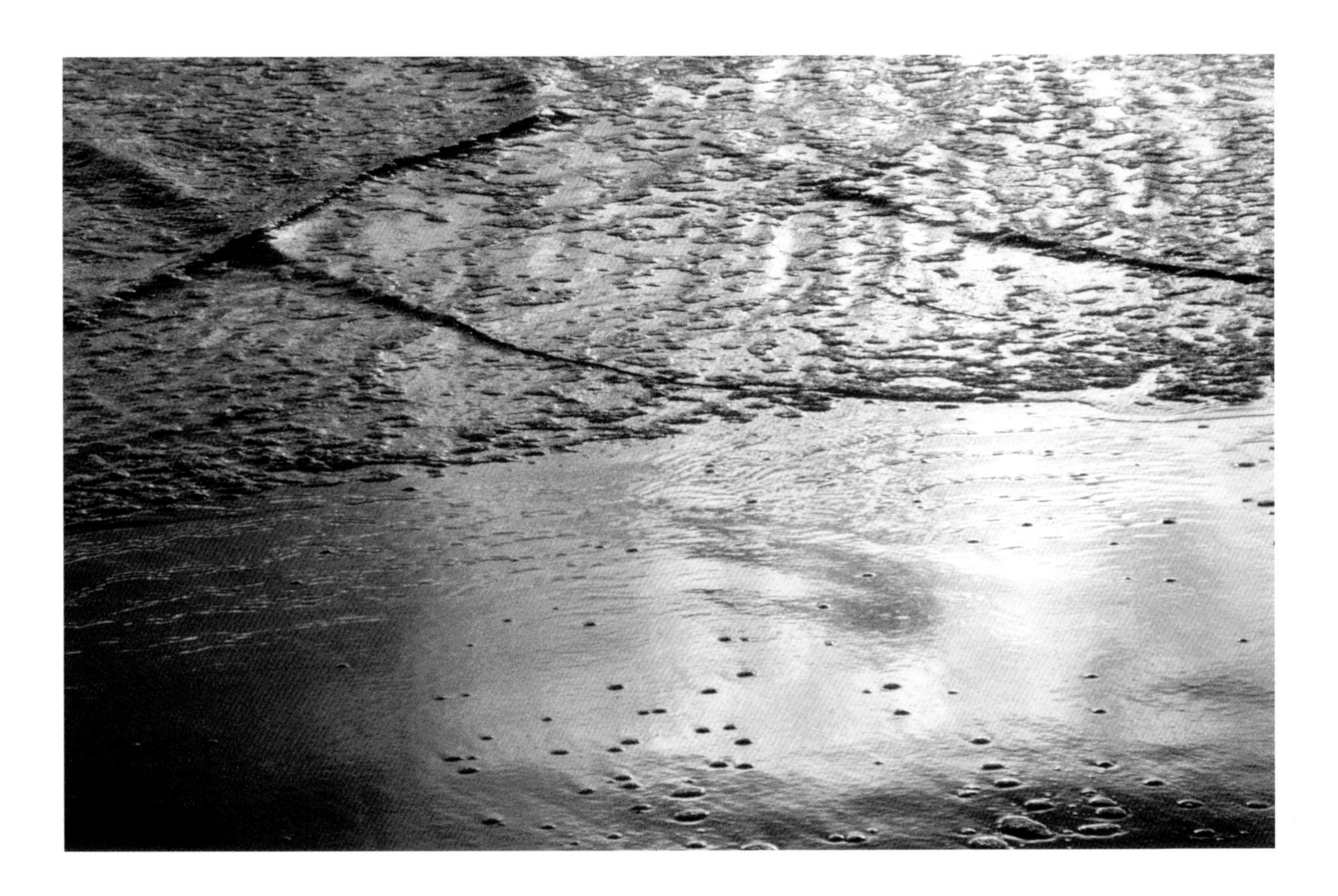

to Julie, Beth and Chris,
whose love and support make
my life meaningful and my
work comprehensible.

roger cooper

IMPRESSIONS

ROGER COOPER | JOHN ERICKSON

Impressions

Cover *Monet Pond,* Northland Arboretum, Brainerd, Minnesota 2000

Page i *Swedish Flag on Dock, Moonlight,* Lake Vonern, Sweden 1997

Page iv *Autumnal Light, Reflected Leaves,* Cannon River, Faribault, Minnesota 1997

Page vi *Dawn, Old Town,* Stockholm, Sweden 1997

Back cover *Leaves and Vines, Doorway,* Carmel-by-the-Sea, California 2001

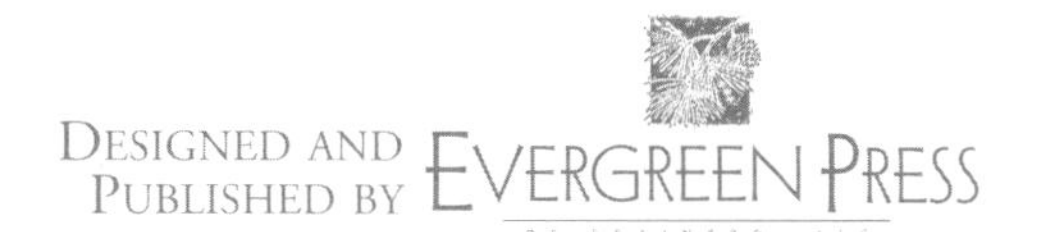

Designed and Published by Evergreen Press

201 West Laurel Street
Brainerd, Minnesota 56401

Printed by Doosan Printing
Seoul, Republic of Korea

ISBN: 0-9661599-5-0

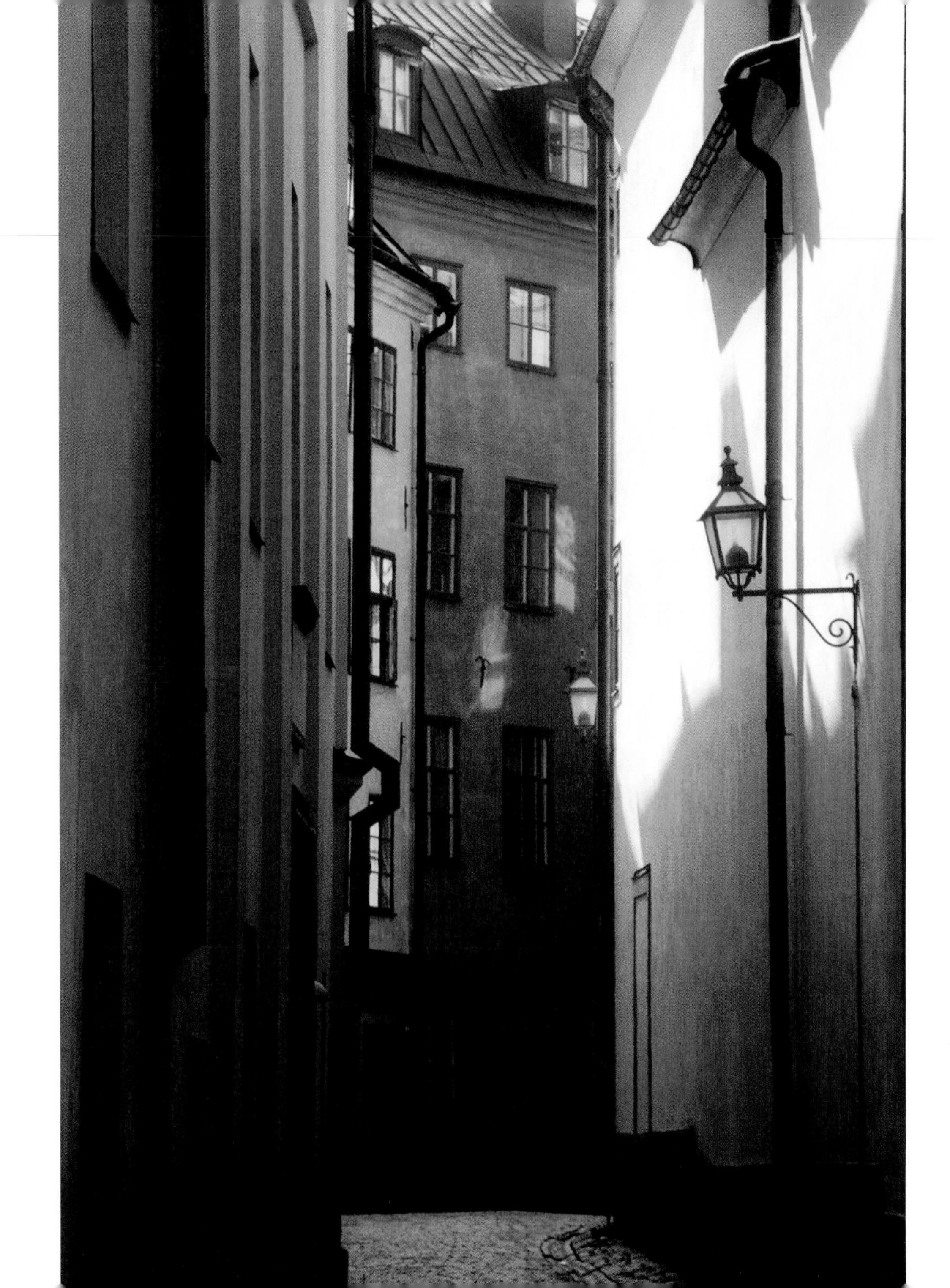

Introduction

The interrelationships between the visual image and the written word have been recognized for a long time, as the aphorisms "a picture is worth a thousand words" and "a poem creates a visual image in one's mind" clearly reveal. This nexus was first explored by the ancient Egyptians, whose craftsmen regarded the visual image of two-dimensional works of art as extensions of their pictographic system of writing. For the ancient Greeks, word and image were vehicles for exploring parallel aesthetic concerns, such as the pregnant moment which dominates both the drama of Sophocles and the visual compositions of the contemporary pediments of the Parthenon. This linkage continued to be explored in the drolleries adorning the pages of *The Medieval Books of Hours,* in Albrecht Dürer's illustrations of episodes of *The Manual of the Christian Soldier,* by Erasmus of Rotterdam, and more recently in Aubrey Beardsley's illustrations of Oscar Wilde's *Salome.*

A detailed study of such synergies would reveal that the visual image in these examples is not merely a banal illustration of the literal meaning of the written word that accompanies it. On the contrary, word and visual image are independent vehicles of aesthetic expression joined to one another for the express purpose of extending the range of aesthetic meanings formulated by the percipient.

IMPRESSIONS must be regarded in the same light. Roger Cooper, poet, and John Erickson, artist, have known each other for five years and have developed an aesthetic rapport. On more than one occasion, that rapport has created opportunities in which John's images were on exhibition at cultural gatherings during which Roger recited his poetry. The logical extension of such synergies was IMPRESSIONS, in which Roger's poems would be paired with John's photographs. In keeping within the traditions of the aesthetic criteria—by which visual images are not mere illustrations of the written word—the juxtaposition of poem and photograph here invites the individual to read the poem and to contemplate the photograph in the hope that a deeper significance will emerge.

I first discovered John's photographs shortly after I moved to Minnesota, when I received an invitation to an opening at a local art gallery. Close-minded about what I would find there, I was initially reluctant to attend, but was goaded to do so by my wife, Anna. To my surprise, but not to Anna's, my eyes were filled with wonderful, visual images. So enthralled were we that, at that very opening, we purchased both *Reflections in Stream,* Kristinehamn, Sweden 1997 (page 106), and *Cartway,* Riverton, Minnesota 1999 (page xiv). *Reflections in Stream* was immediately framed and installed in our living room, where it shared pride of place with other original works of art by American Abstract Expressionists and ancient *objets d'art* from our private collection.

To appreciate the richness and variety of John's approach to visual elements in his photographs, one must first understand that John regards photography as "writing with light." One must, therefore, be particularly sensitive to the effects of light on the portrayed images. Light reacts to a lens as to a human retina, causing color and form to register either on film or in the mind. That reaction may reveal a spectrum of colors, the complete reflection of light or its complete absorption. John's photographs, therefore, are often orchestrations of either polychromy

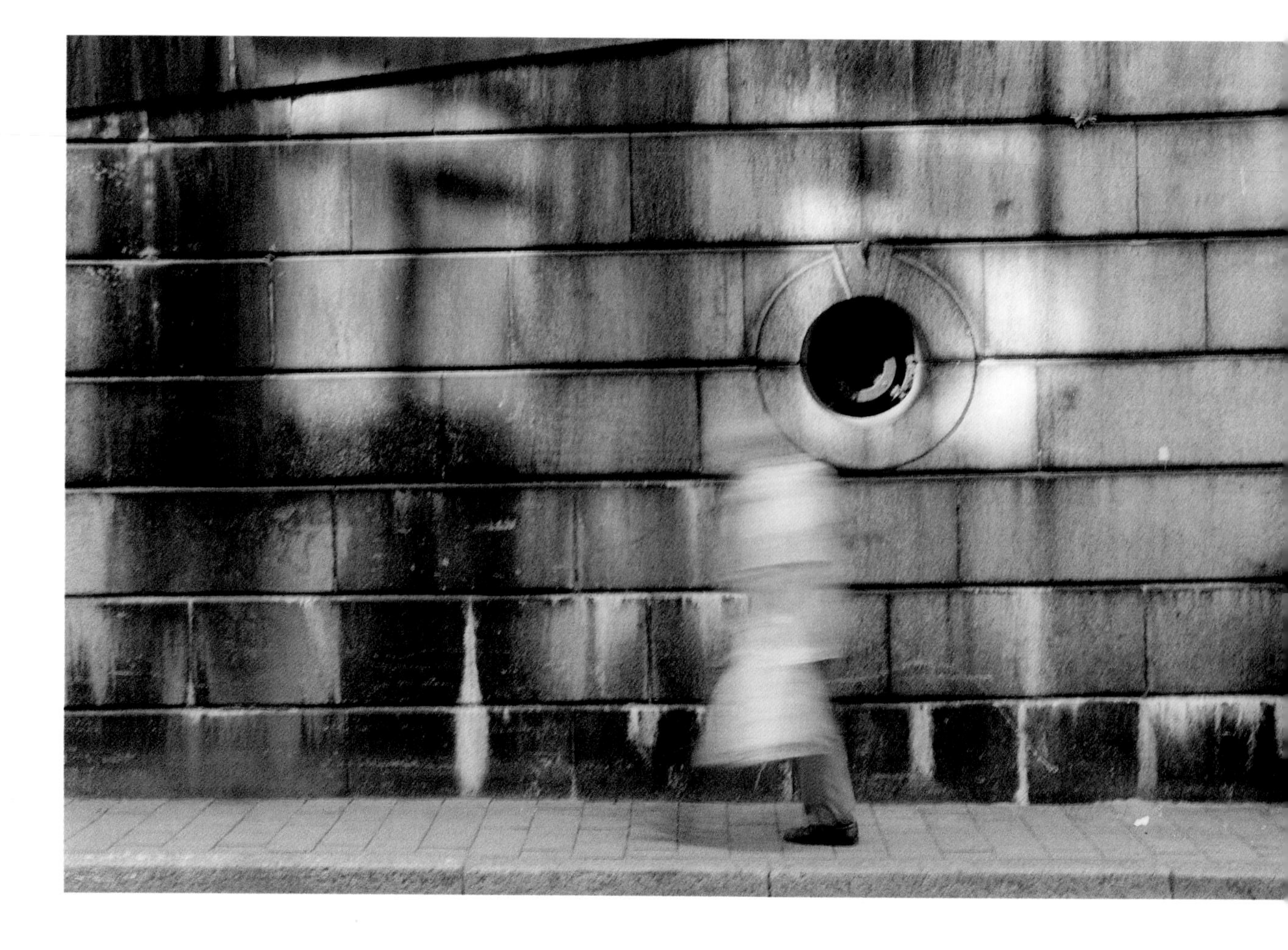

Woman Walking, Old Town, Stockholm, Sweden 1997

Family Crypt, Uppsala Cathedral, Uppsala, Sweden 1997

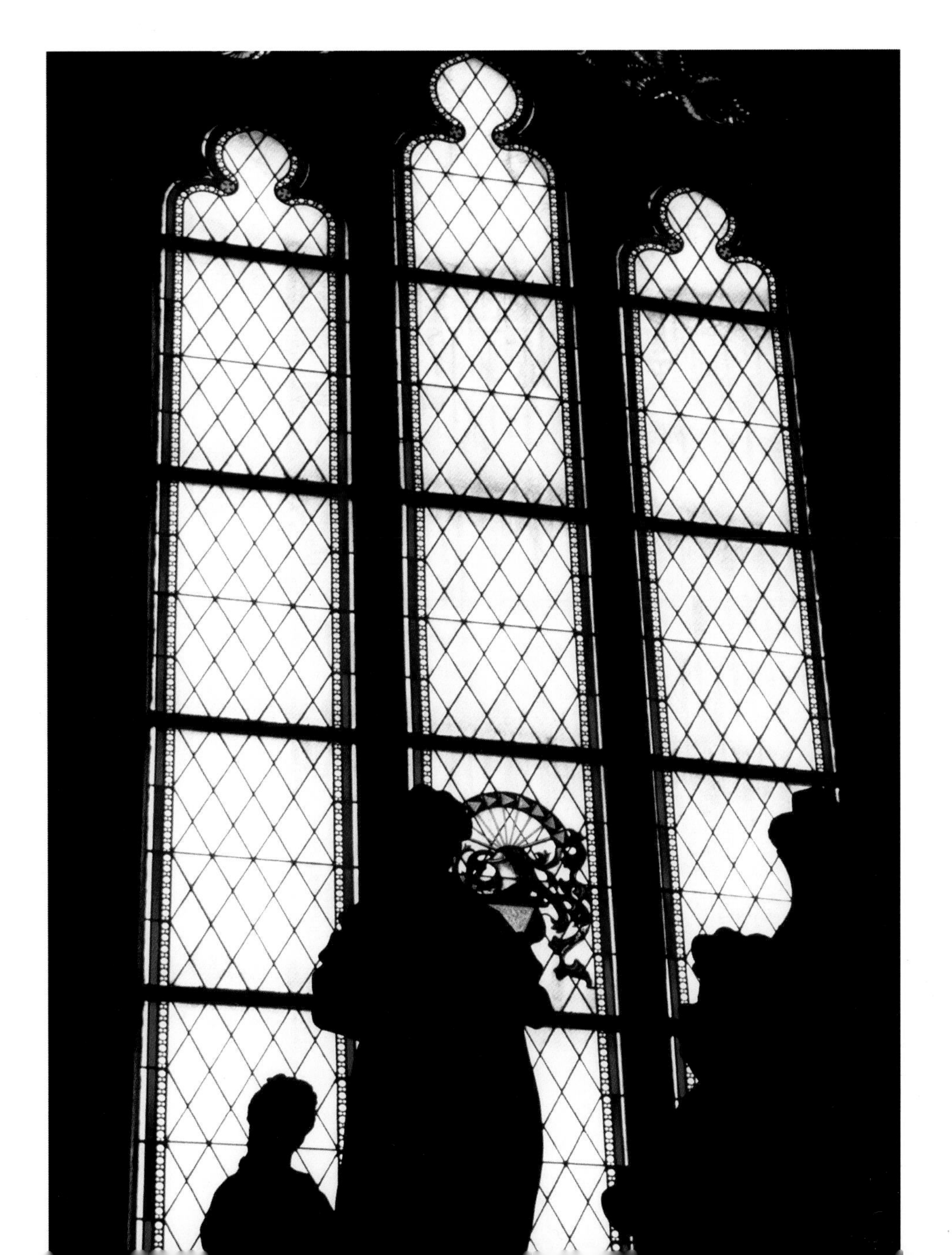

(*Beyond One Lifetime*, Corcoran Art Gallery, Washington, D.C. 2000, page 16) or monochromy. Monochromatic themes include *Carolus Linnaeus,* Uppsala Universitet, Uppsala, Sweden 1997 (page 74), in which values inherent in hues of white are masterfully explored, as well as in his silhouette series *(Statuary,* Capitol Grounds, Des Moines, Iowa 1993, page 42), which likewise reveal nuances permeating what is generally perceived to be a monolithic black shadow.

John's manipulation of light results in a series of what I term "color fields," echoing attainments in painting. The more familiar of these are his landscapes *(Field at Dawn,* Near New Prague, Minnesota 1997, page 58), some of which capture a mystic horizon similar to those employed by abstract expressionists, such as Stamos or Rothko *(Couple at Sunset,* Carmel Beach, Carmel-by-the-Sea, California 2001, page 69 and *Line, From*

Clumper's Point, Gull Lake, Minnesota, 1998, page 81), John's use of light to create chromatic effects is inextricably linked to his sensitivity to form, the second component of a visual image. When composing, John captures the nuances of design inherent in Nature or in man-made objects, transforming the realism of the visual elements into powerful abstractions. This characteristic is evident in his ability to capture the crackled effect of asphalt *(Figure,* St. Paul, Minnesota 1998, page 25), the varied appearance of ice *(Winter Light,* Mississippi River, Brainerd, Minnesota 1997, page 45), and the subtleties of the water, either on surfaces *(Reflections in Stream,* Kristinehamn, Sweden 1997, page 106) or as movement *(Sunlight in Waterfall,* FDR Memorial, Washington, D.C. 2000, page 41). On occasion, these aesthetic concerns virtually mask reality *(On Toe, Tornstrom Auditorium,* Brainerd, Minnesota 1995, page 38).

Tree, Wetlands, Brainerd, Minnesota 1996

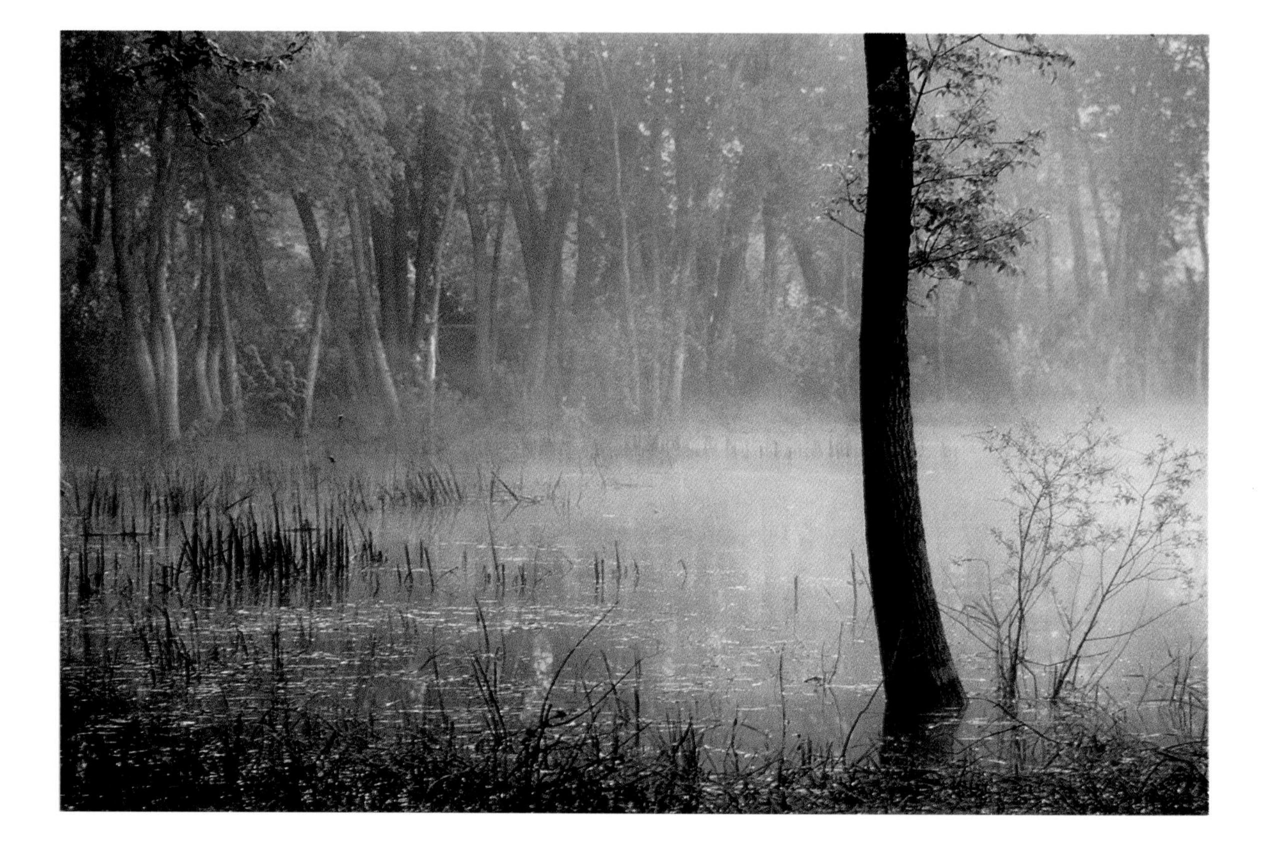

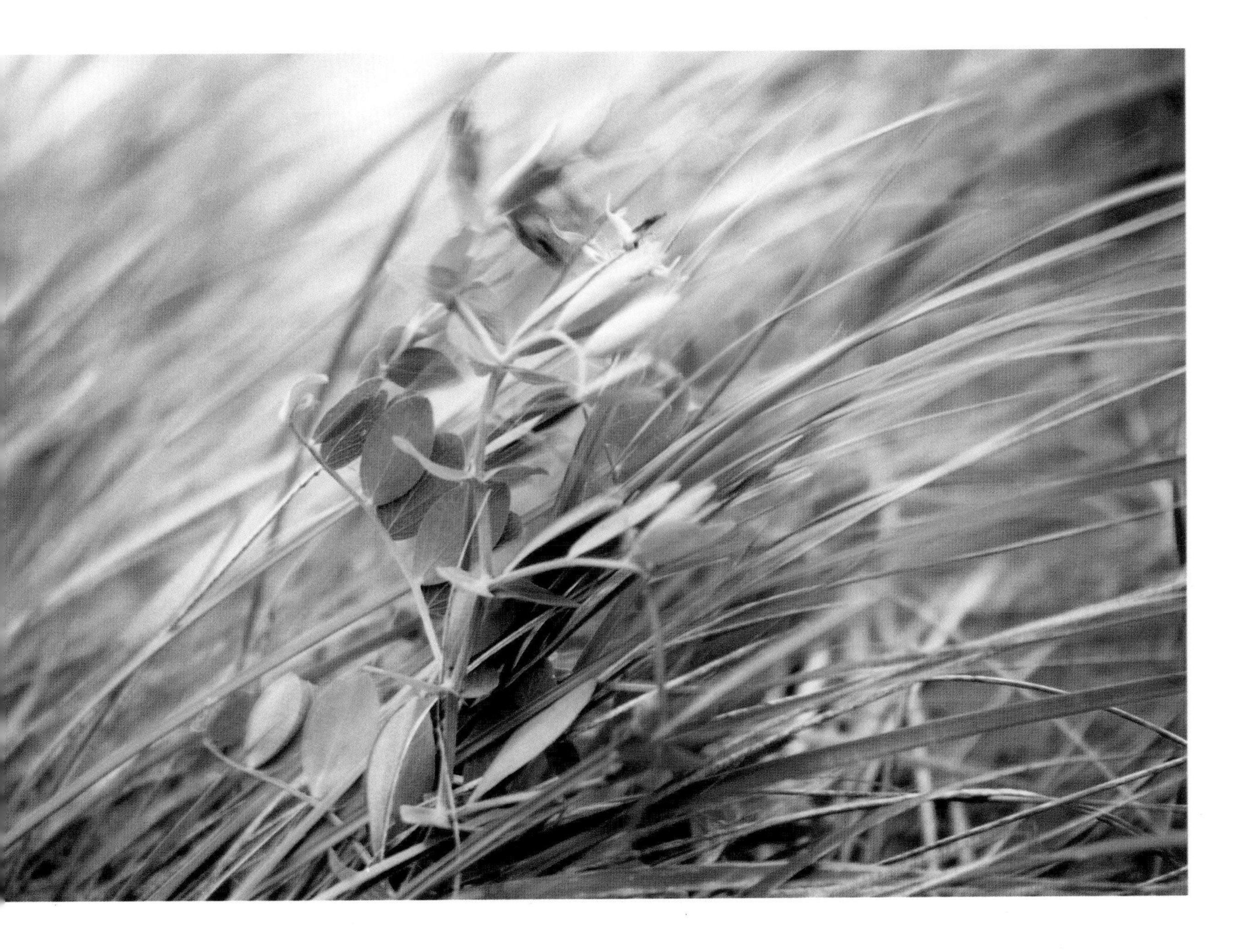

Lake Superior Wildflower, Sand Dune, Park Point, Duluth, Minnesota 1996

Light not only creates a visual form of color on retina or lens, but also its own, independent image, particularly evident in John's cast shadows series, such as *Woman Walking, Old Town,* Stockholm, Sweden 1997 (page viii) and *Dawn, Old Town,* Stockholm, Sweden 1997 (page vi).

Among light's characteristics is its ability to create images that suggest how transitory and ephemeral Nature can be, as seen, for example, in the waves of grain in *Lake's Edge,* Rice County, Minnesota 1998 (page 23)—the soft-focus of which also connotes how supple and soft Nature can be, as in *Exit from 210,* Aitkin County, Minnesota 1995 (page 52) and *Infinity,* Big Sur, California 2001 (page 88).

My acquaintance with Roger, a fairly new-founded one, derives from John's invitation to both Anna and me to join John in one of those cultural opportunities at which John's photographs were on exhibition while Roger recited his poetry. As soon as Roger took the podium and began to recite, I realized that his delivery, perhaps honed from his experience as a Lutheran clergyman, was informal, yet authoritative, and utterly engaging. I leaned forward, perched on the edge of my seat, as Roger deliverd "Coming to Grips with Constantine" (page 19), a poem awash with meaning about peace and religion in the aftermath of 9/11. Anna and I could not help but reach out and clasp our hands during Roger's recitation of "Turn Out the Light" (page 109). So compelling was its message for two career-driven individuals that we seized the opportunity to take home a copy of that poem, distributed at the end of the evening, after which we had it framed and placed it in our study as a reminder to step back and "absorb the peace."

The themes of Roger's poetry are redolent with expressions of the human condition. One can conveniently divide these expressions into four major thematic

Butchart Gardens, Resurrection, Victoria, British Columbia 1995

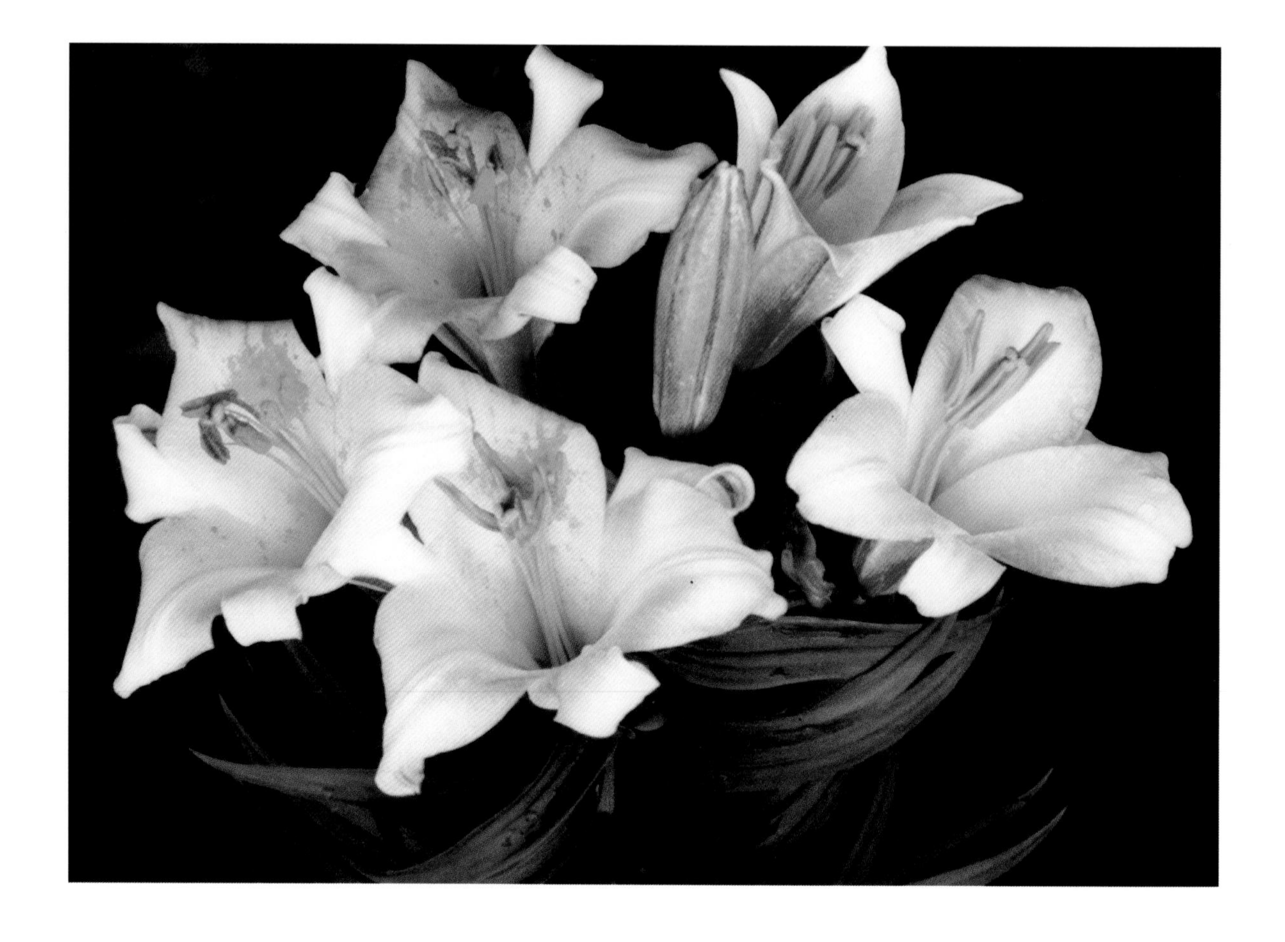

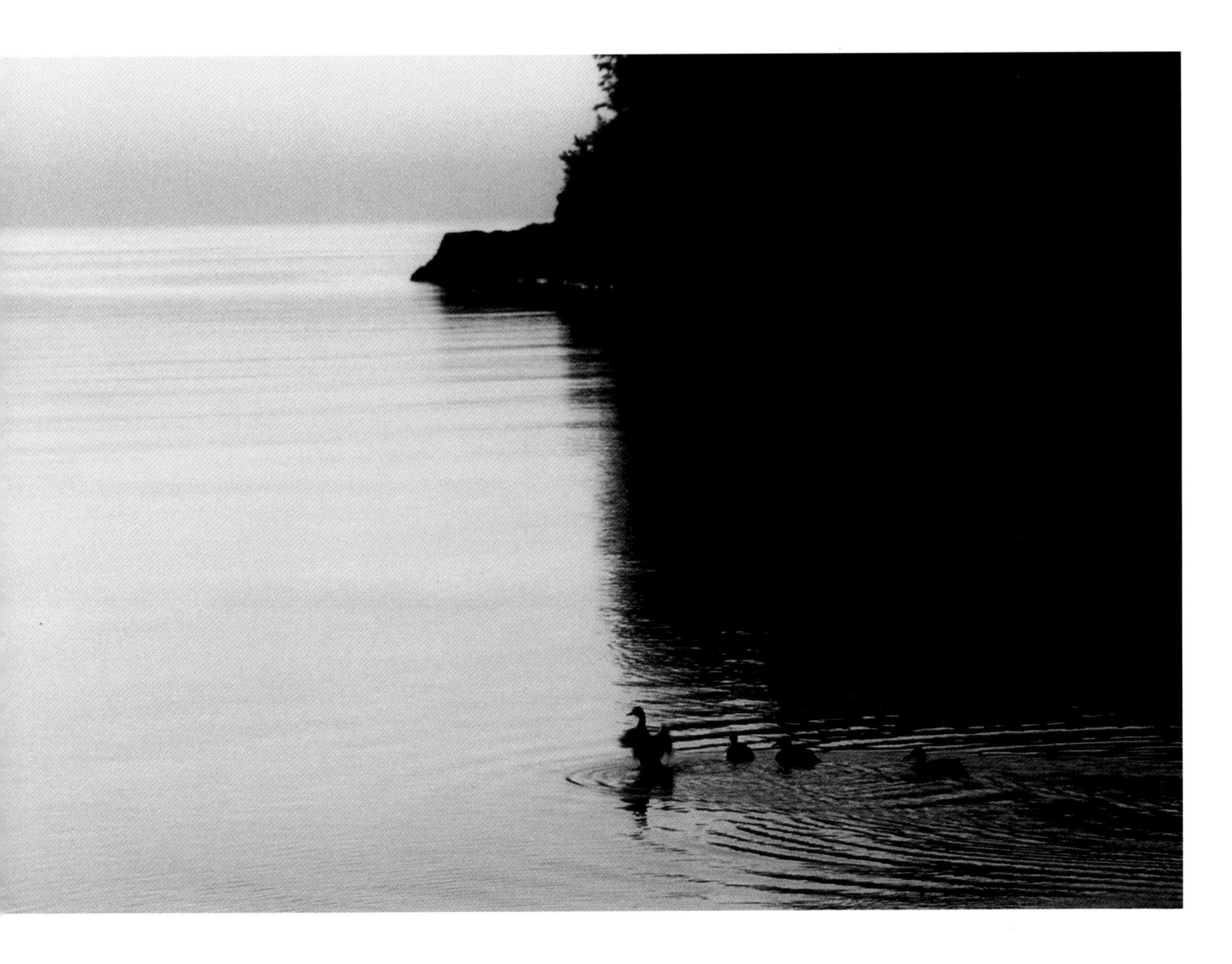

Arising, Flood Bay, Near Two Harbors, Minnesota 1999

categories—Pain (and Death), Conflict, Forces, and Isolation—although a careful reading of all suggests a unitarian approach explored via the polyvalence of interlocking meanings. "Coming to Grips with Constantine" (page 19), an exemplar of the theme of Conflict, reveals that personal decisions are not always easy to reach and that, oftentimes, one must live with uncertainty. And uncertainty is part of the human condition, as are themes explored in Pain and Death. In these, Roger is concerned with conflict, but here examines ways in which an individual, either in isolation or under a spiritual, one might say divine, force relates to the cosmos in order to gain a deeper understanding of self. It is characteristic of Roger's thematic venturings that Pain, Death and Conflict reveal despair, but that, too, there is always hope: Optimism is a viable option.

The themes addressed in Pain and Conflict may justly be regarded as belonging to a dialectic which informs the poems dealing with subjects of Forces and Isolation. Although each poem here is an independent, stand-alone composition, the ensemble provides a rich exegesis for self examination. The Forces of Nature embodied in these poems—"Lake Waves," "Lake Ice," "The Wind," "Warm Air," and "Today's Rain"—are transformed, becoming multi-faceted images defining the human condition. These poems are subtly optimistic. Their issues are successfully resolved, as if the hand of a deity were at work. The poems grouped together under themes of Isolation explore the events operative upon individuals relative to the societal collective and allude to processes of integration or separatism. The personae of these poems appear to be possessed of a degree of free will which contrasts with the divine pre-determination perceptible

Cartway, Riverton, Minnesota 1999

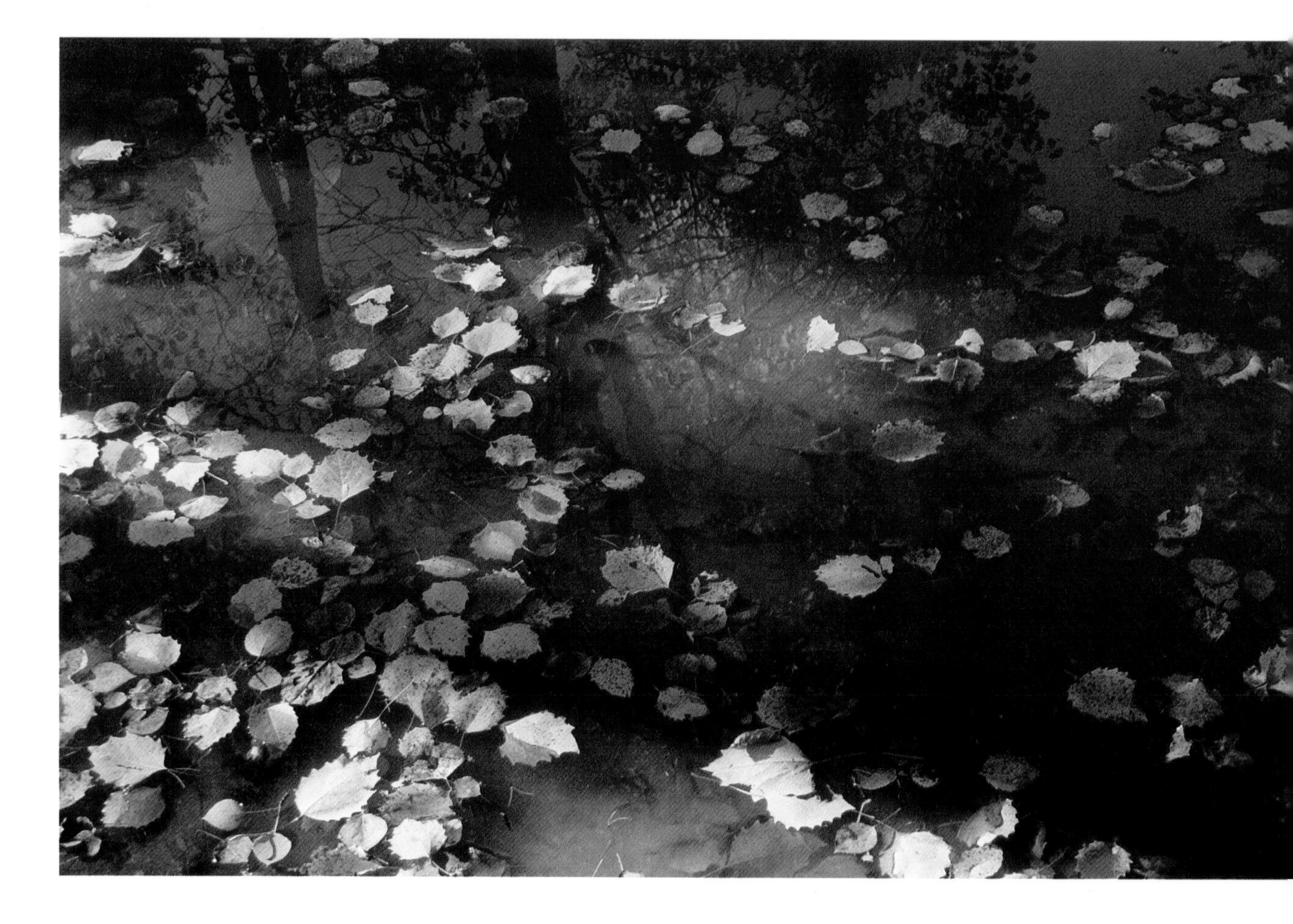

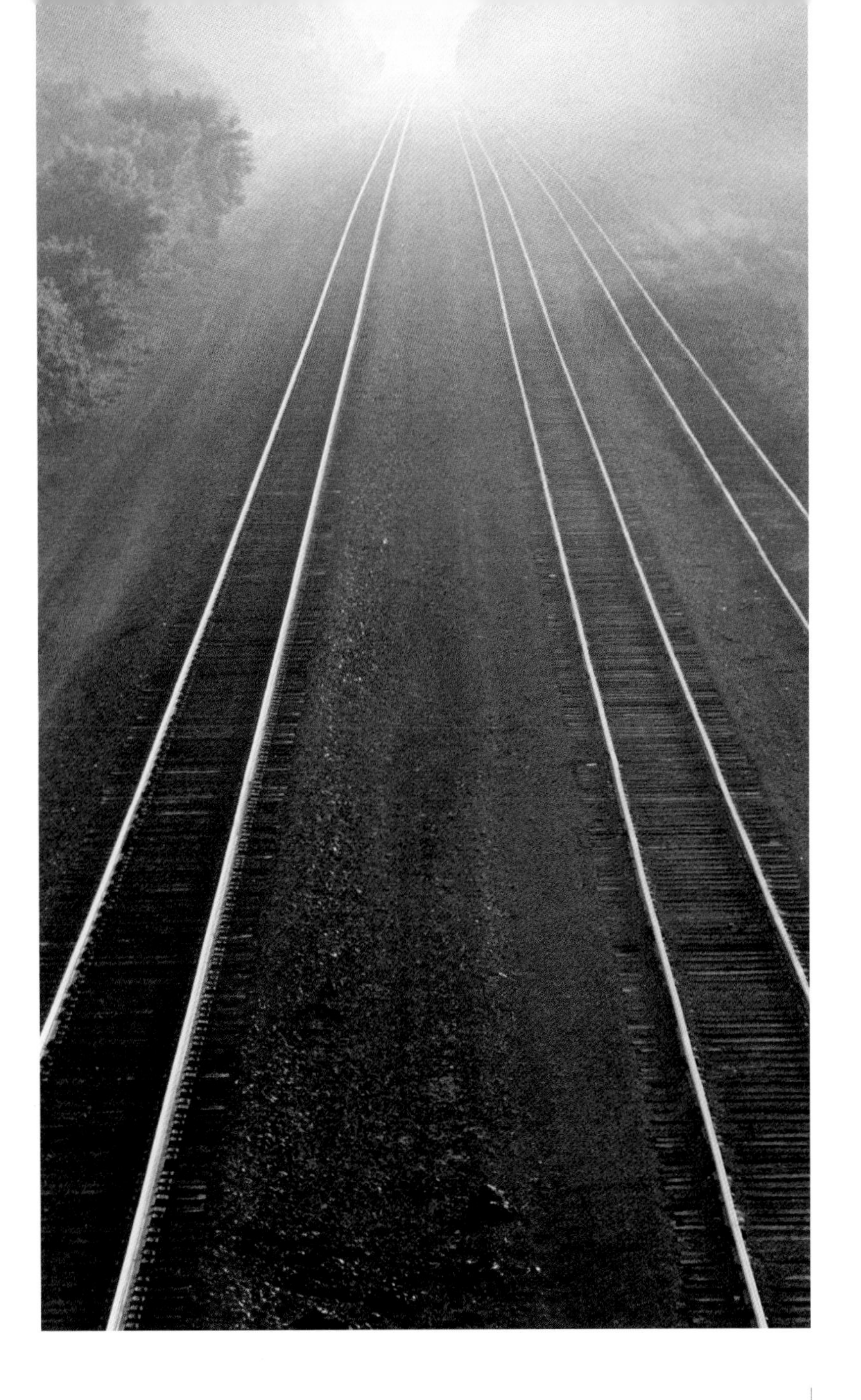

Infinity, Brainerd, Minnesota 1998

in Forces. Because of this intended dialectic between free will and pre-destination, the poems of Forces and those of Isolation are possessed of a deeper interpretative significance than each poem would possess on its own.

The pairing of Roger's poems and John's photographs in IMPRESSIONS can, therefore, only be regarded as a successful synergy: Author and artist not only understand an individual's integration into the great scheme of Nature's divine design, but also articulate that integration with printed word and creative image. In so doing, the pairing of poem and photograph opens up a picture window onto the world of human experience and, thus, exposes all of its subtleties, thereby permitting the percipient a greater opportunity of understanding one's self.

Dr. Robert Steven Bianchi
Baxter, Minnesota
January 2002

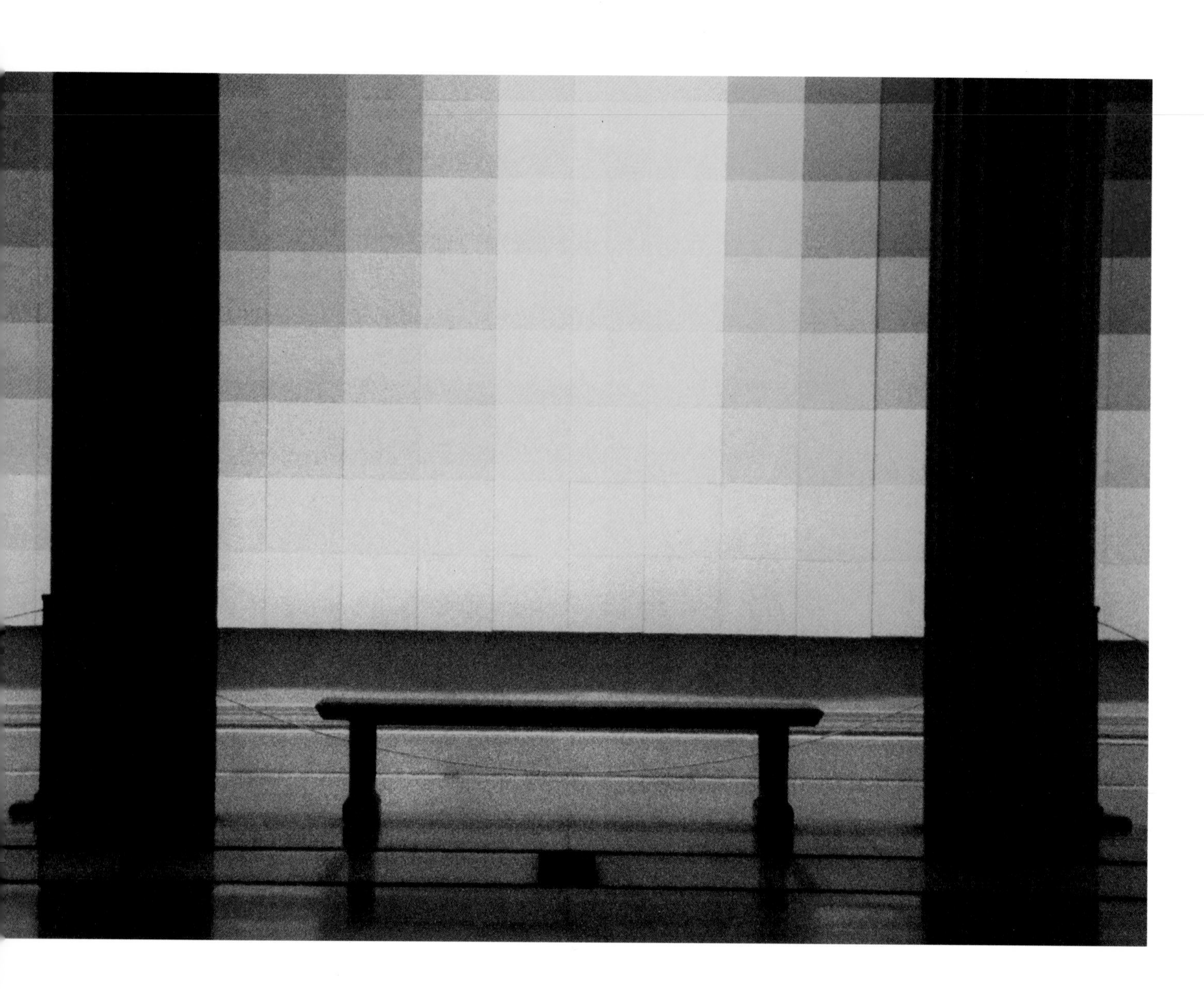

A painting or a poem
Reflects a part of life,
Beyond one lifetime.

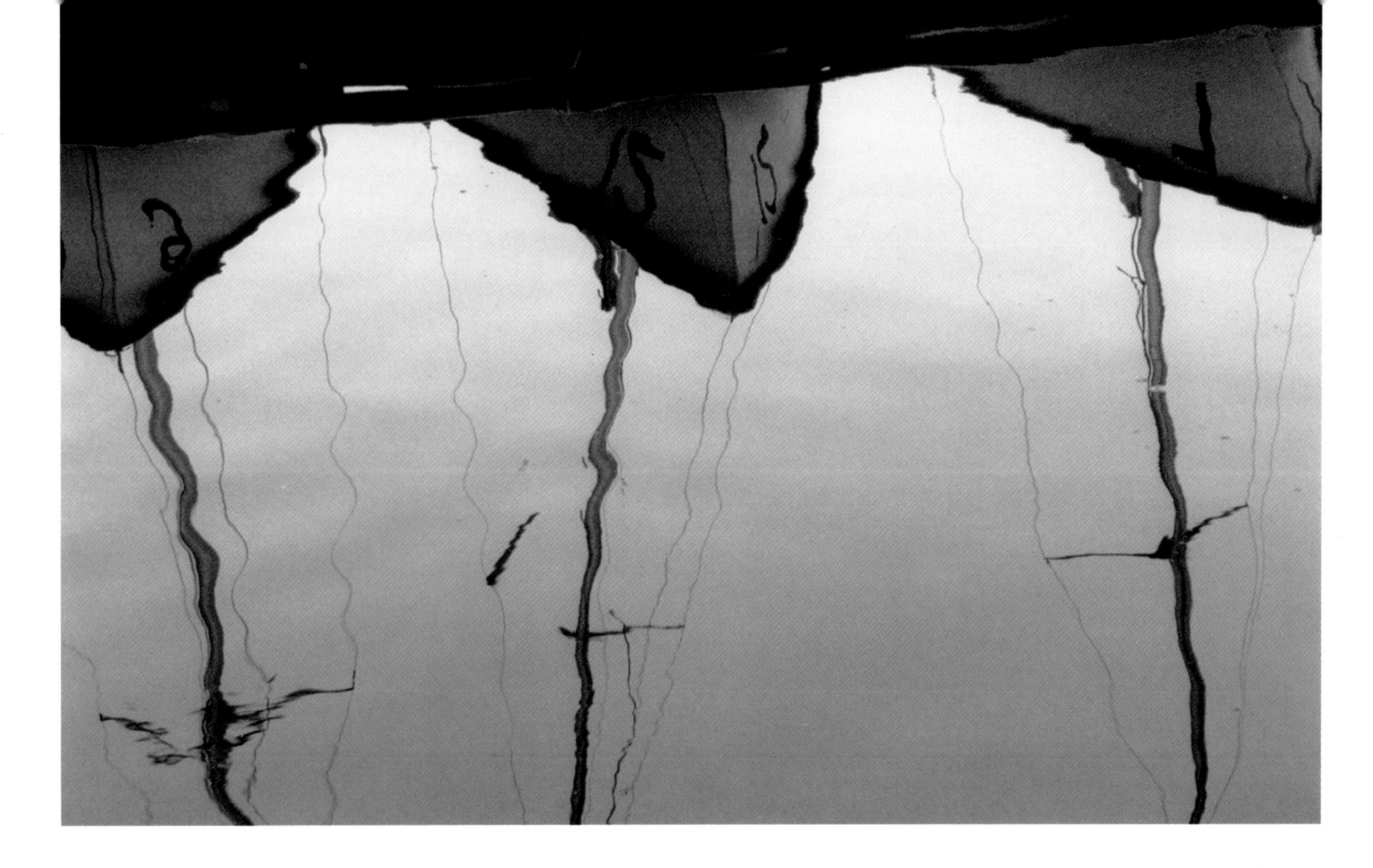

A quiet rhythm moves the boats
brushing against each other in the night.
At sunup they will move out, away from each other,
at different speeds, in different directions.
As the ocean begins to receive the sun,
they wander back in twos or threes,
beckoned, beckoning, ready to rest.
Mooring lines are loose, not tight,
allowing them to rise and fall with tugs of tides.

10/20/71

Boats at Dawn, Mystic River, Mystic, Connecticut 1998

State and Church, City Hall and Cathedral, Stockholm, Sweden 1997 | 04/25/97

After the battle of the Milvian Bridge,
Constantine thanked Jesus.

His empire was secure
From armed enemies.

But,
At some level
He knew
He needed more.
He needed *them.*
The bishops came to Nicea,
Walking along the lake,
Coming from everywhere,
Summoned by the Emperor.
They went inside
Between armed guards,
Political police,
Who wouldn't let them out
Until they agreed.

The bishops walked in,
They could not walk out,
What else could they do?

They had to agree
Or they could die.
Right there.

They voted on the truth
And created a standard statement
To be the rule,
For measuring
The truth
And loyalty.

What could they do?
More than one
Honest argument,
Reasoned opinion
Disappeared
In ignominy.

What could they do?
He fed them well,
They slept as they could;
They ate and argued
According to someone else's schedule.

They had to agree.
They were outposts of empire.

They had to agree.
They were divining the will of God;
The consensus of bishops;
Norma normans;
Peace for a time.
Peace for a place.
Peace for a person.

At the battle of the Milvian Bridge:
Who won?
Who lost?
What?

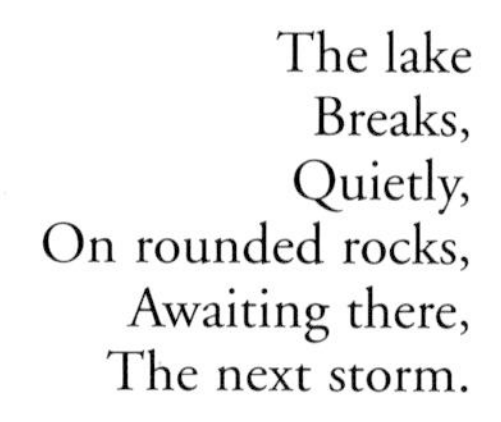

The lake
Breaks,
Quietly,
On rounded rocks,
Awaiting there,
The next storm.

Lone eagle
Drops from birch branch,
Shattering
The glassy calm
Of our lake.

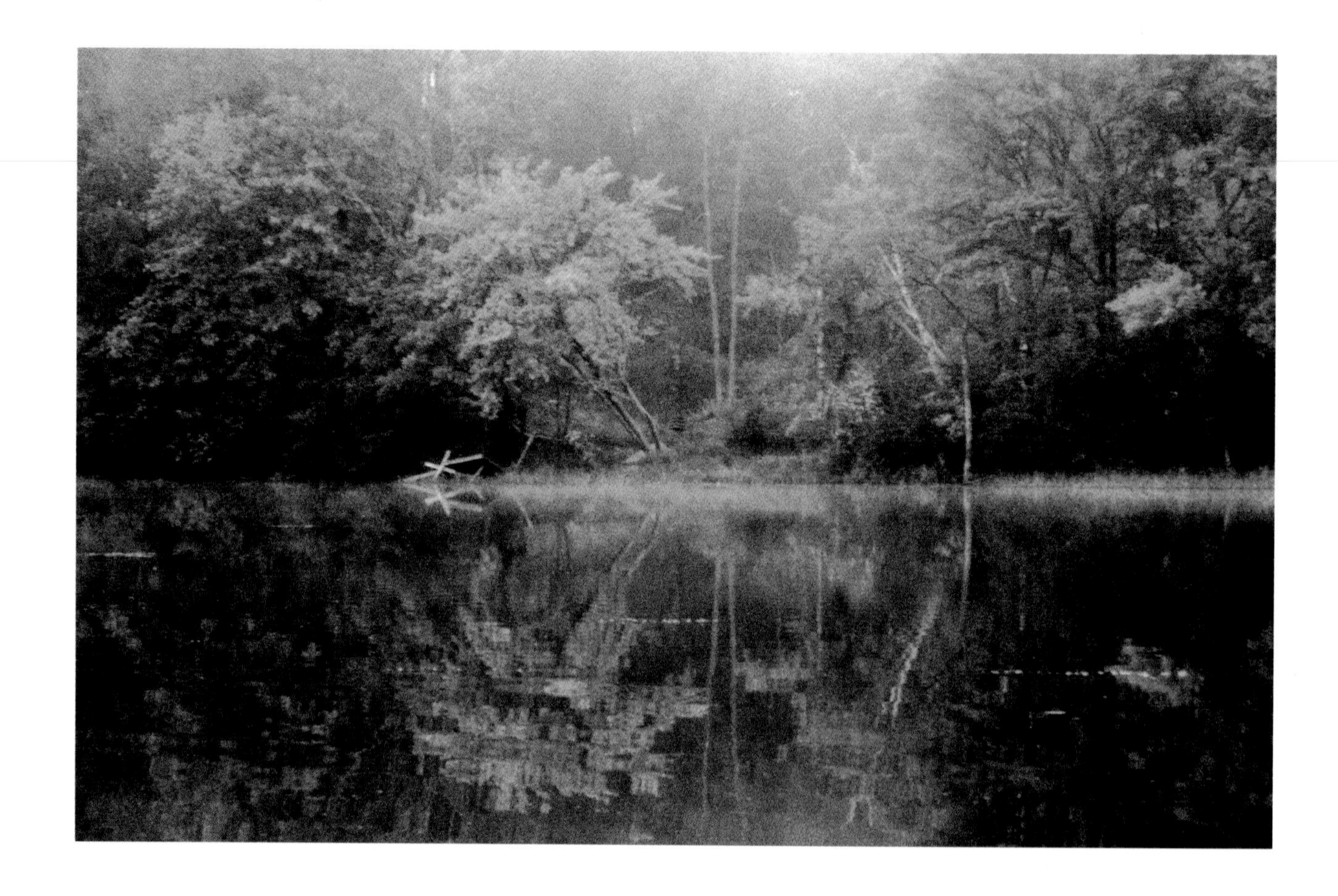

07/02/98 | *Bay of Retreat,* Mississippi River, South of Riverton, Minnesota 1996

LATE FALL:
Shivering,
Ice emerges all at once,
From shore to shore.

LATE WINTER:
Lengthening,
Long grey days
Stir fish,
Moving them
From the bottom up.

LATE SPRING:
Eroding,
Ice melts,
From the edges in,
Warmth nibbling at its waxy edges.

LATE SUMMER:
Blowing,
Strong storms
Tear off water weeds,
Moving them quickly,
Downwind.

A mid-life crisis
Becomes a course correction,
If you face the pain.

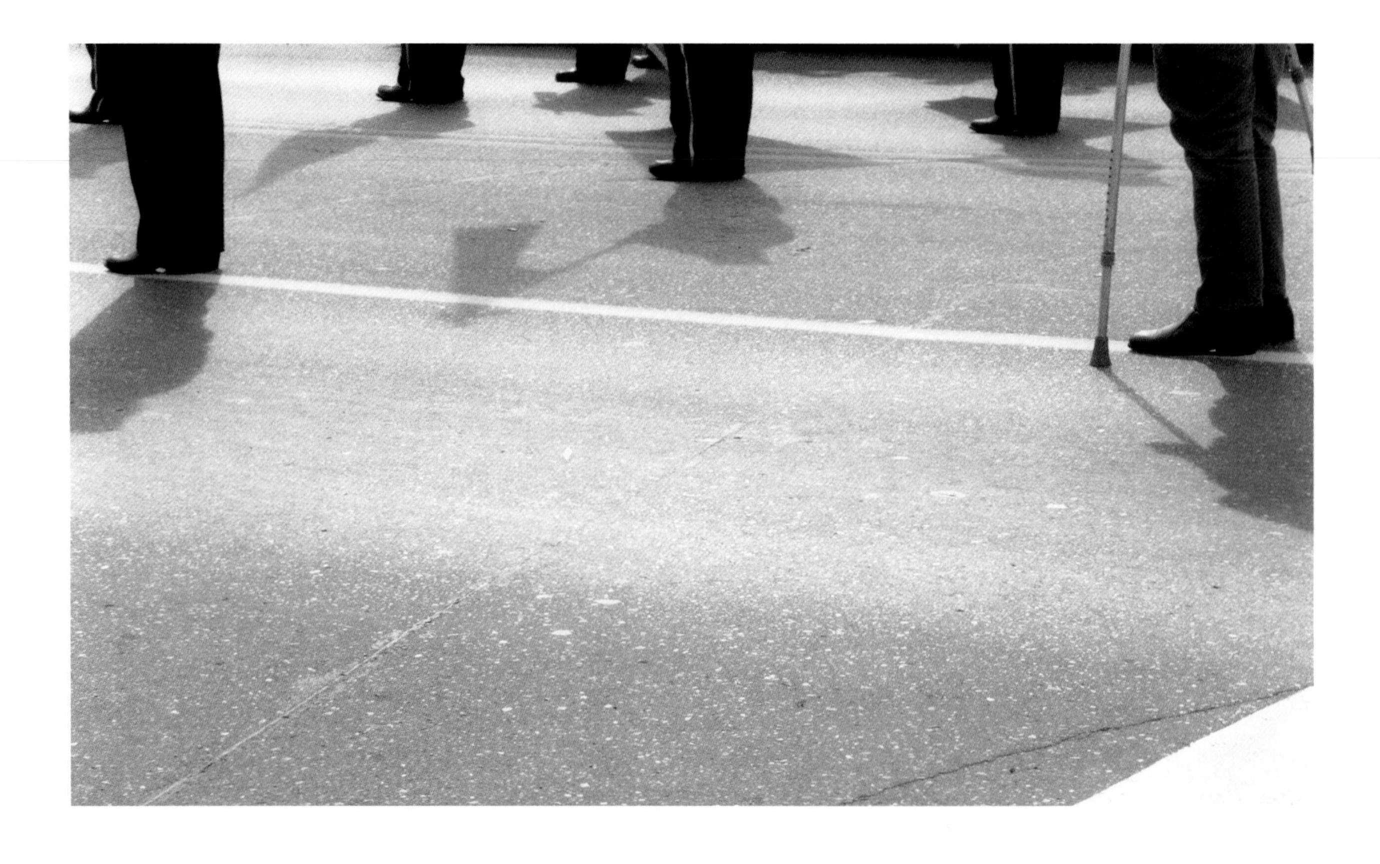

06/06/01

Color Guard, Parade, Walker, Minnesota 1998

For amber waves of grain:

Remember raves of pain
When teeth or ears
Ached
Unceasingly,
When your side hurt
And you walked to school
Sweating,
Bent over,
The sure signs of appendicitis.

But can you,
In any way,
Know another's pain?

We are cut down
Like wheat,
Ready or not,
Abruptly,
Into emptiness.

We draw our nourishment
From earth;
Dying,
We return that gift.

What we leave behind,
The husks,
The hulls,
The chaff of everything we do
Is scattered by the wind.

And life,
And death,
Begin
Again.

This end of the lake
Is quiet now.
Deer are browsing silently.
A solitary junco,
Chirping from a bough,
Evokes a memory,
A long lost ache.

Tree Branch, Turtle Lake, Minnesota 1998 | 04/28/97

I caught a glimpse of you
Passing by,
On the other side
Of the road.

Only an instant,
Time for a glancing look,
A flash through the window
Was all it took
To remind me
Of everything
You mean to me.

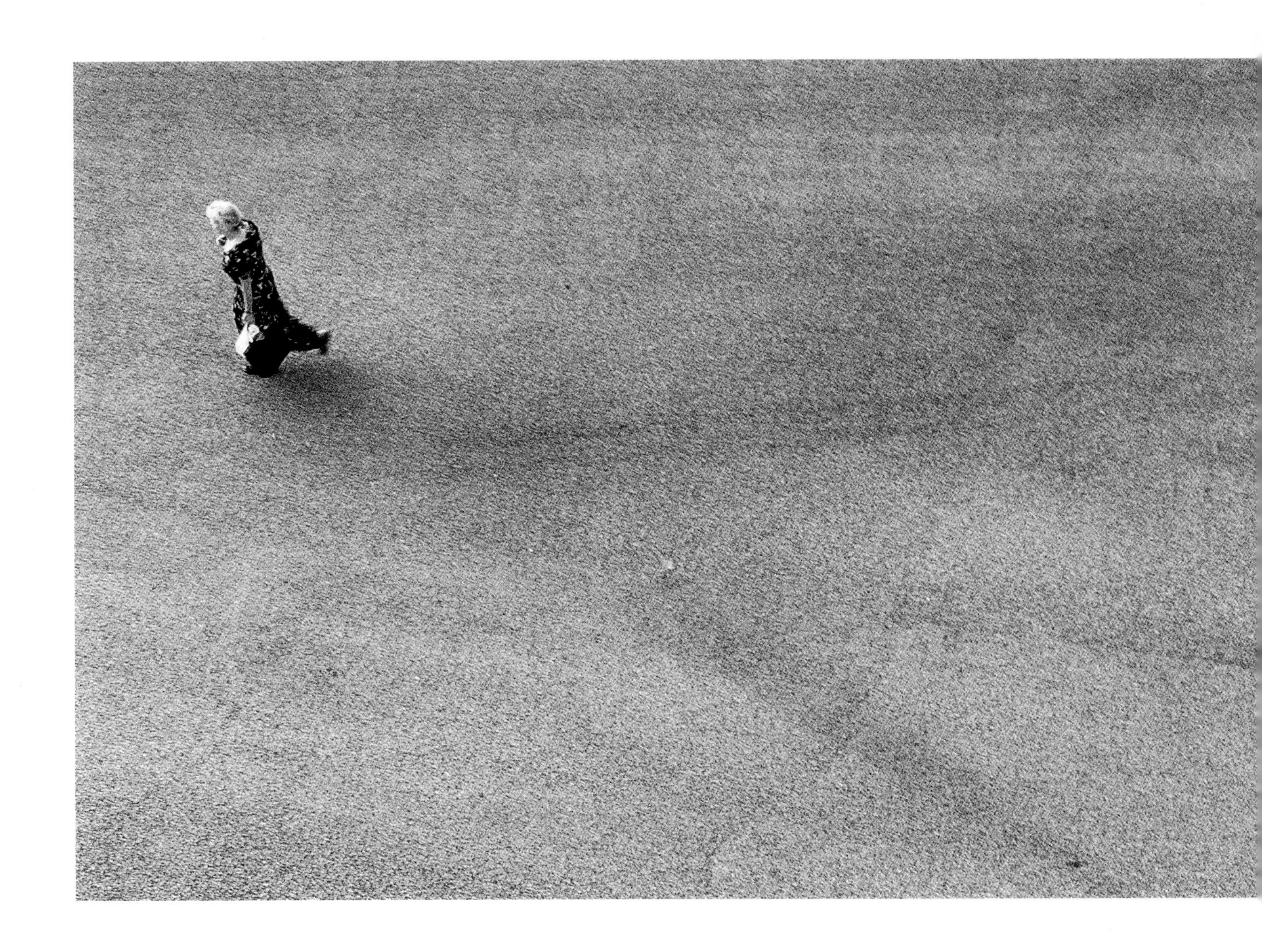

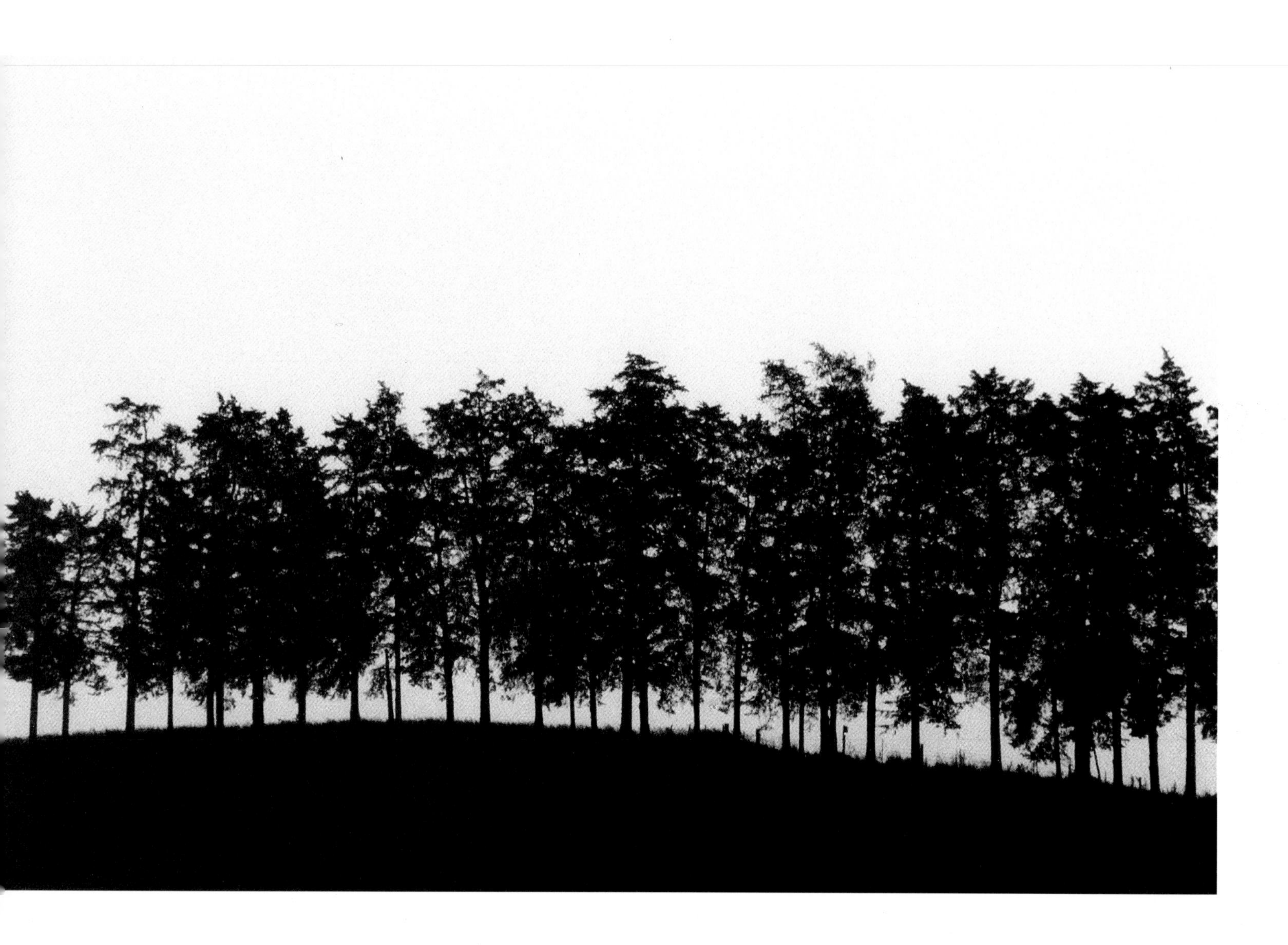

I did not see
That line of trees
Along the hill
Until today.

Against the southern sky
They stand,
Stretching grey and spiking green,
They seem to be
A curtain
Waiting to receive
A moment
To be seen.

Spring
Is this time
Between long lake snows
And thunder blundering storms,
When tiny trout snuggle under grass
And big clouds bloom
In millpond reflections.

You saw me once,
A young girl
Bright and waiting
To be found.
So much changes,
In so little time!

Lively juices
Evaporate,
Until the slightest
memory
Remains.

The slow sun
Warms the marble,
Grass,
And sand.

A few frogs waken
From their sleep,
Aware,
But unaware,
Of where they are.

And you
Are here,
Again,
With me,
Looking at that line of
trees,
Along the hill,
Waiting to be seen.

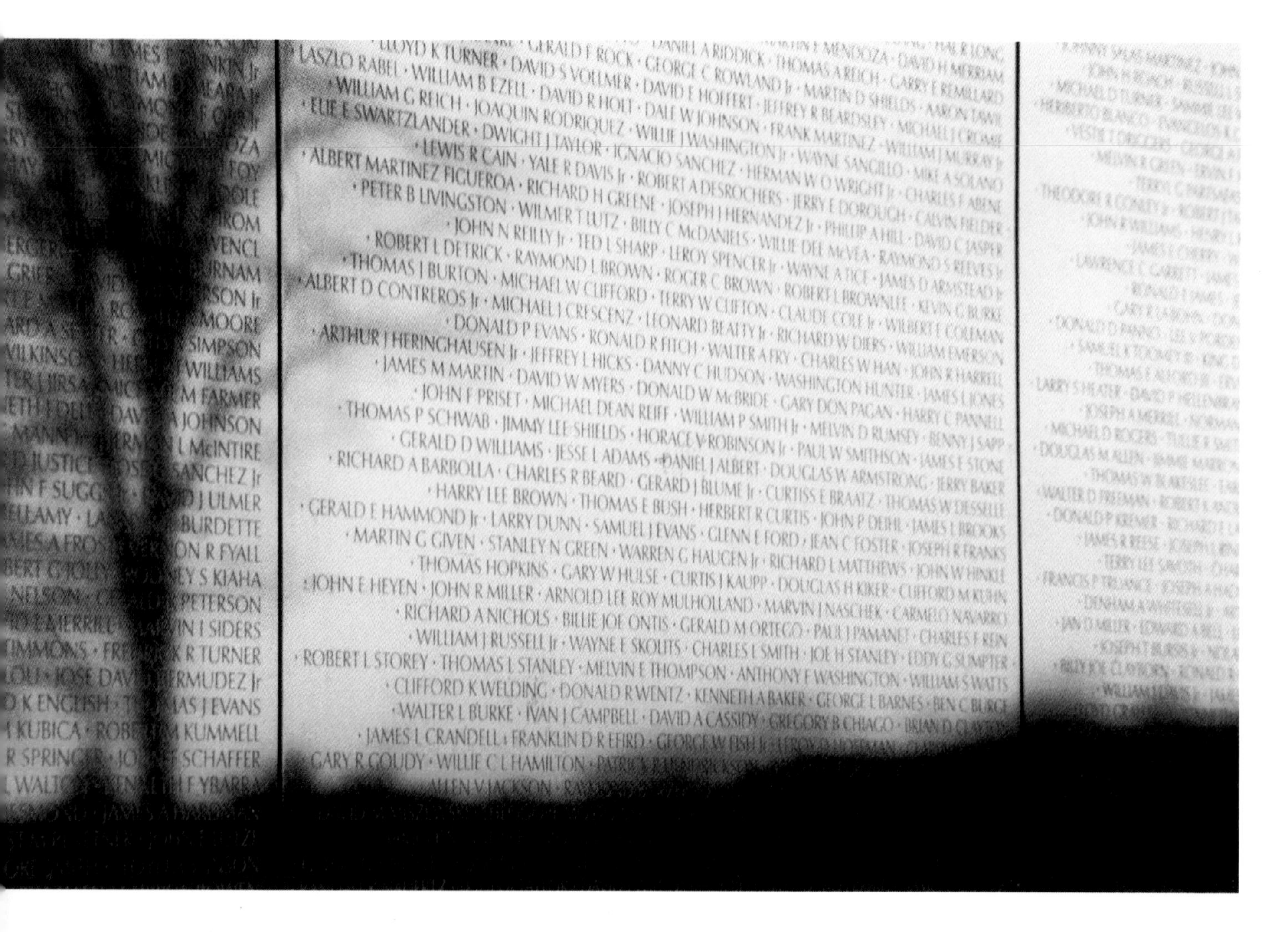

I have another chance
To reflect
The glory
Back to God
Which emerges in my mind
And in the warmth of my hands.

Each heartbeat
Has a power,
A stillness
In the flow of tiny bits of matter
Forming and reforming,
Making me a mirror
Of the universe
Or multiverse.

I am a part
Of all that is,
The solid,
Dense,
And emptiness
My mind arranges in my eyes and ears
Within the frame of time,
The fragmented mirror of experience.

And God is seen in part,
As if,
And when
I see your eyes
Reflecting me
In mine.

Known to God, Vietnam Memorial, Washington, D.C. 2000

11/02/90

Mourning the death
Of a shared dream,
Pain is dissolved
In torrents of tears.

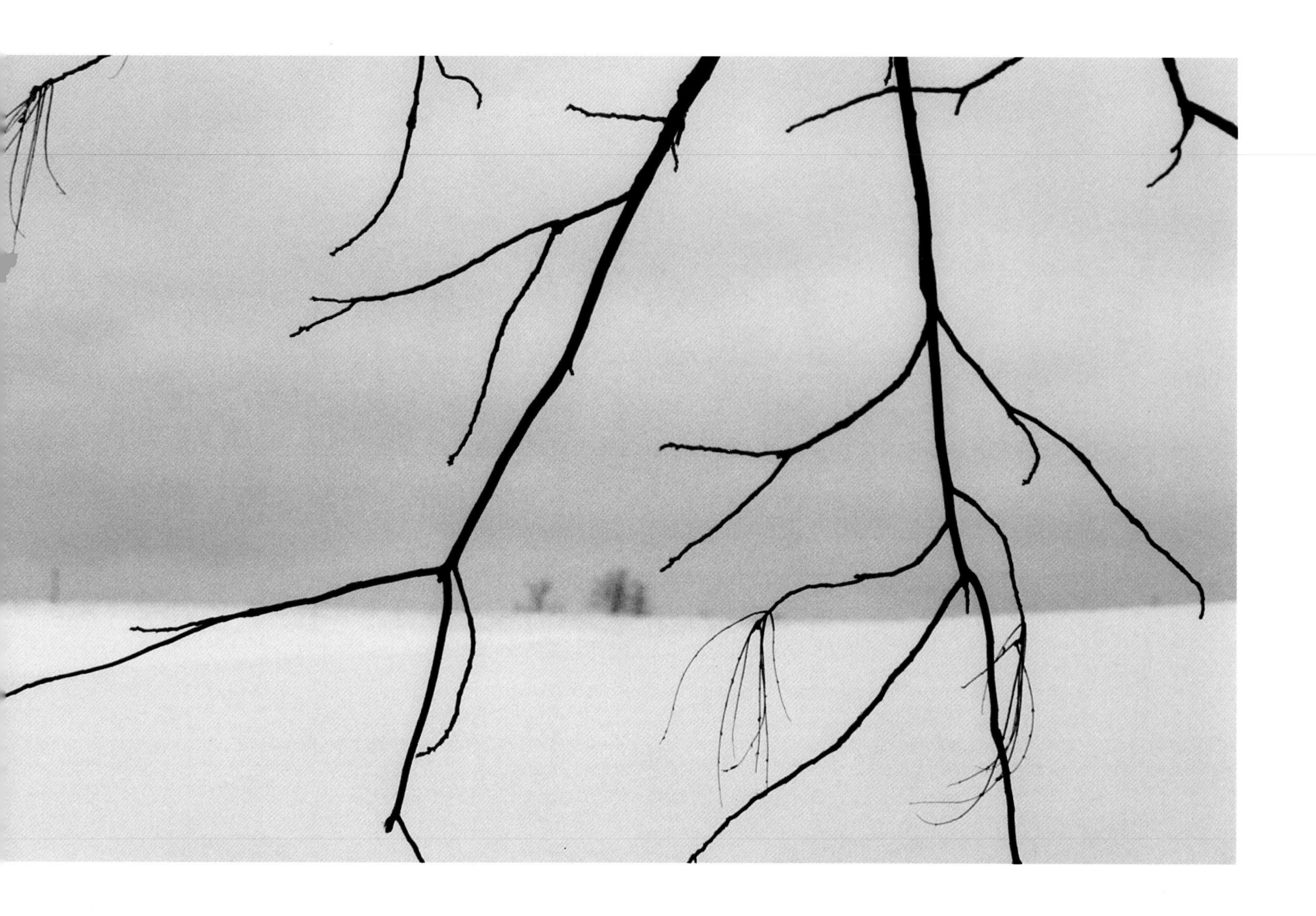

Branches and Distant Trees, Winter, Breezy Point, Minnesota 1993

03/15/70

Morninglight greys curtainfolds long
before the Winterday begins.
Salmonsun on greensky polishes pearl
clouds after Winterday has gone.
The western houses expand black
among bare branches
Except for tiny triangles of light,
framed by arbitrary twigs.

Northwind shakes the lakes and trees,
riffles the nearly clean green river
beneath and beyond the bridge.
Cut and crippled cornstalks point from
earthrise cracking and sealing
at its doubleroot.
Thickened cloudshreds rush southward
under contrails moving north.
Shearing airmass turns in turmoil about
a wing-tearing, roller bearing,
grinding clouds into snow at mid-March.

Snow at mid-March, the dangerous last
gasp whiplash of Winter's storm
tracks moving north, reluctantly,
Chills the tender tips of tulips teased
by warm sun into breaking
brownclods into shade earth.
Red from bloody birth beneath the thin
frostline formed by Winter's finger,
They stiffen as the chill wind bites
their tented pointed sprouts.

I sit, waiting at the window, searching
the sky for some sign of the
cold weight rising.
No birds or dogs go past and children
hurry indoors from the bus,
Placing footsteps beside, inside the
tire tracks in the cold snow.
Occasional descending planes bomb
the valley floor with icy
knifesliced slabs of sound
Around the blossom blasts of
readjusted thrust,
Adding only to the darkness of the snow.

Tulips lined by multilayer skin and cell,
snow and earth, water and root,
reverberate with all the cosmic
changes centered here.
Someone's sun absorbed the energy lately
sprung from brown bulbs,
Irrepressible forces moving earth and
stone, the paradigm of birth, making
life face life in spite of cold and snow.

There will be no other Spring, cold,
dead, immovable.
Summer has its cold, and deadness too.
Fall has its insulating frosts.
Winter has its warming snow.
Snow at mid-March has its will to kill
all blossoming possibilities.

For hope to live, one reflective flower
is enough.

Da-Sein,
Being-There,
Is all there is
Of what we are,
And,
It's enough!

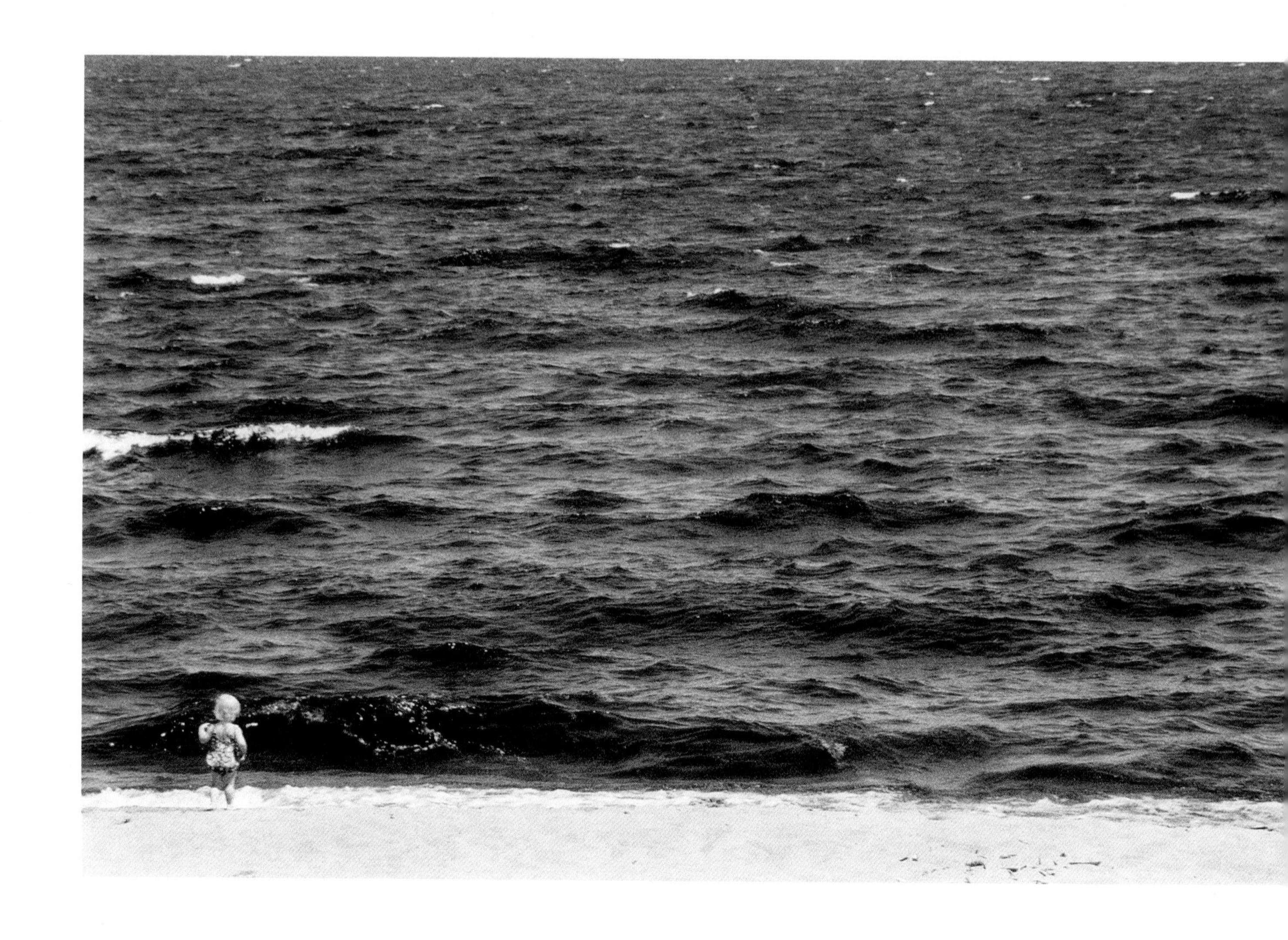

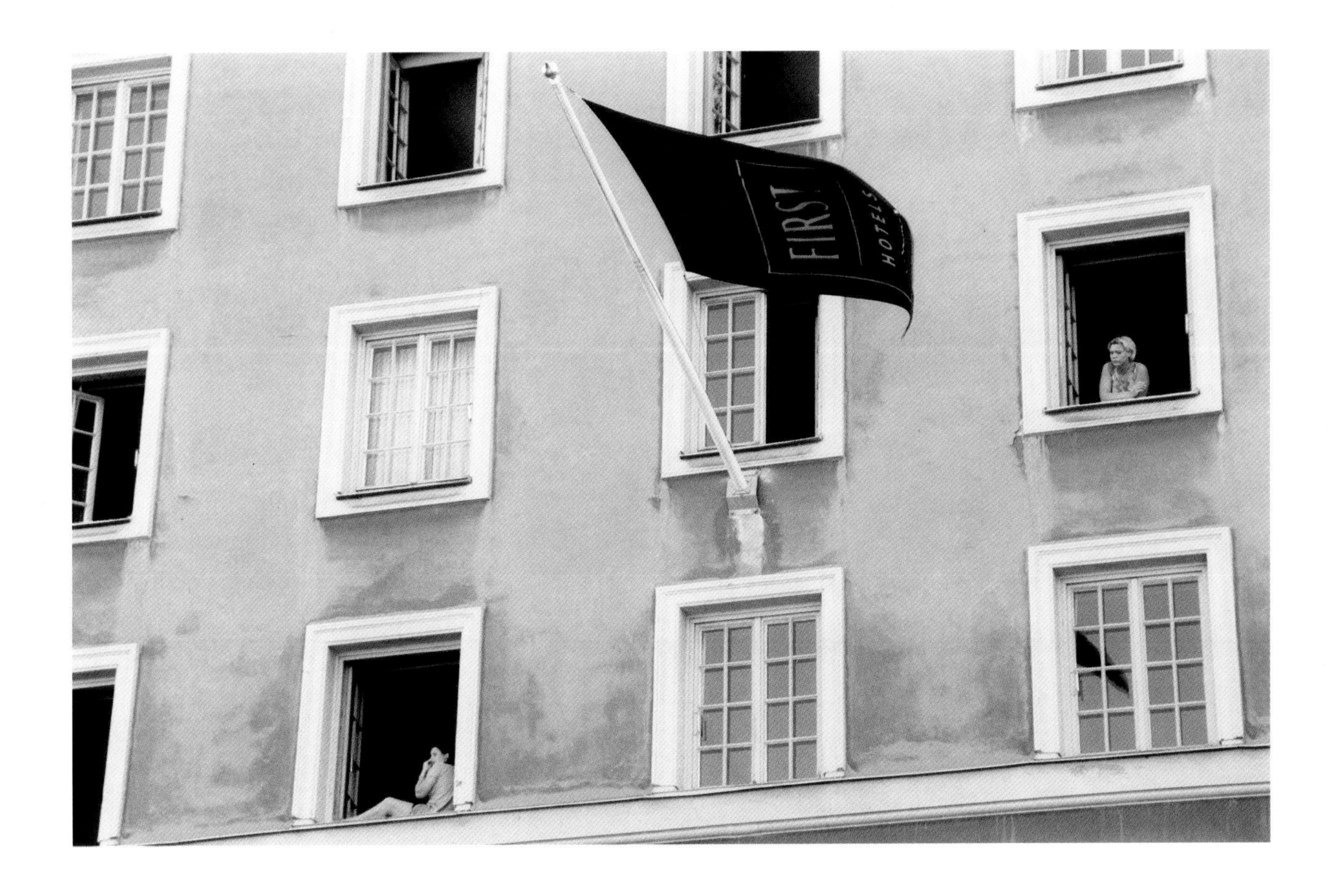

I reach out;
Nothing returns,
Sometimes.

While I wait,
I sometimes wonder
If my reaching
Doesn't matter
More than the sparkle
On the snow.

Hotel Dwellers, Stockholm, Sweden 1997 | 03/15/97

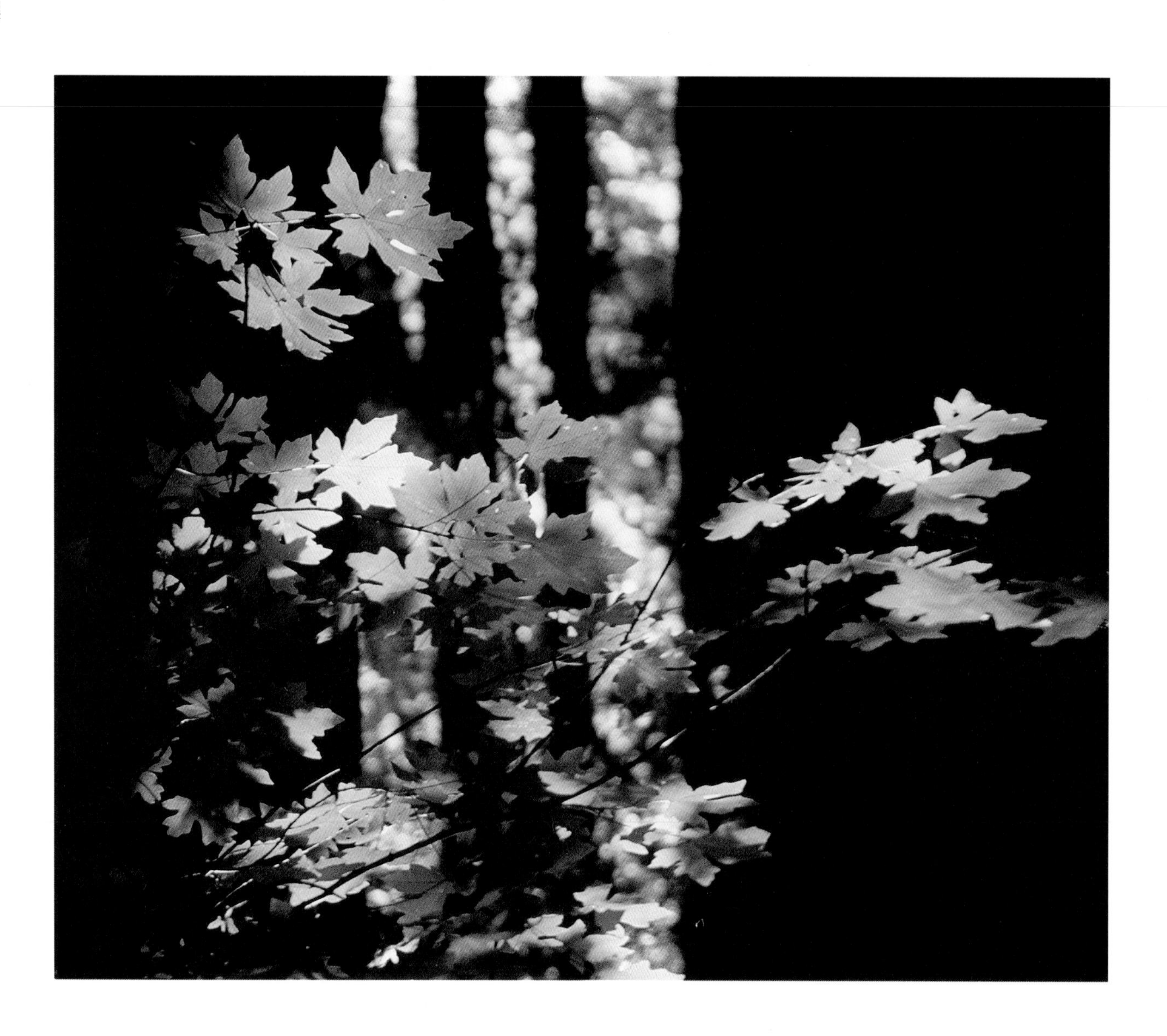

Snow sublimates,
Disappears,
Without a trace.

The woods seem full of life
And energy,
But all the spaces
Between the trees
Are all ways empty.

Sunlight is invisible
Until a leaf,
A branch,
A tree
Gets in the way.

The empty dark
Never really goes away.
It just stays hidden
Every day.

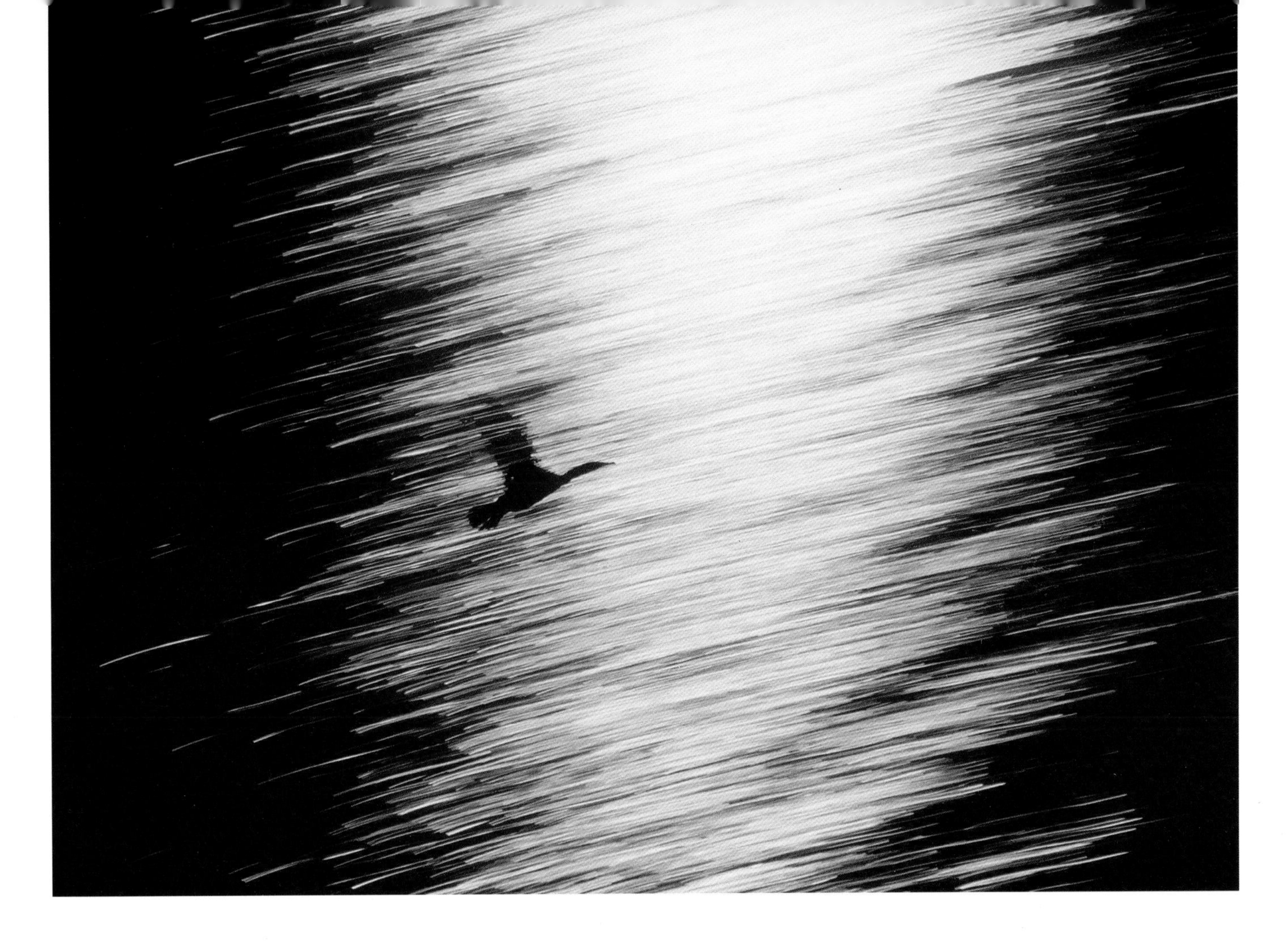

The birds are perched
Along lines and trees,
Afraid to fly,
And so am I.

03/07/82

Bird in Flight, Against the Charles River, Boston, Massachusetts 1998

I spend the testing time testing:

thought against pain
pain against perception
perception against hope
hope against fantasy
fantasy against reality
reality against dream
dream against thought
thought against pain,
again.

Fatigue is my blanket;
Fear my pillow.
Dreams assemble occasional sounds
Into perceptive images,
Arresting my attention.

An excursion into this awful emptiness
yields a desert's painted,
lifeless treasure.

Fossilized memories,
Agatized replacements of reminiscenses,
Concentric growth rings in fallen,
fractured slabs.

09/08/70

Early Morning, Mississippi River, St. Paul, Minnesota 1996

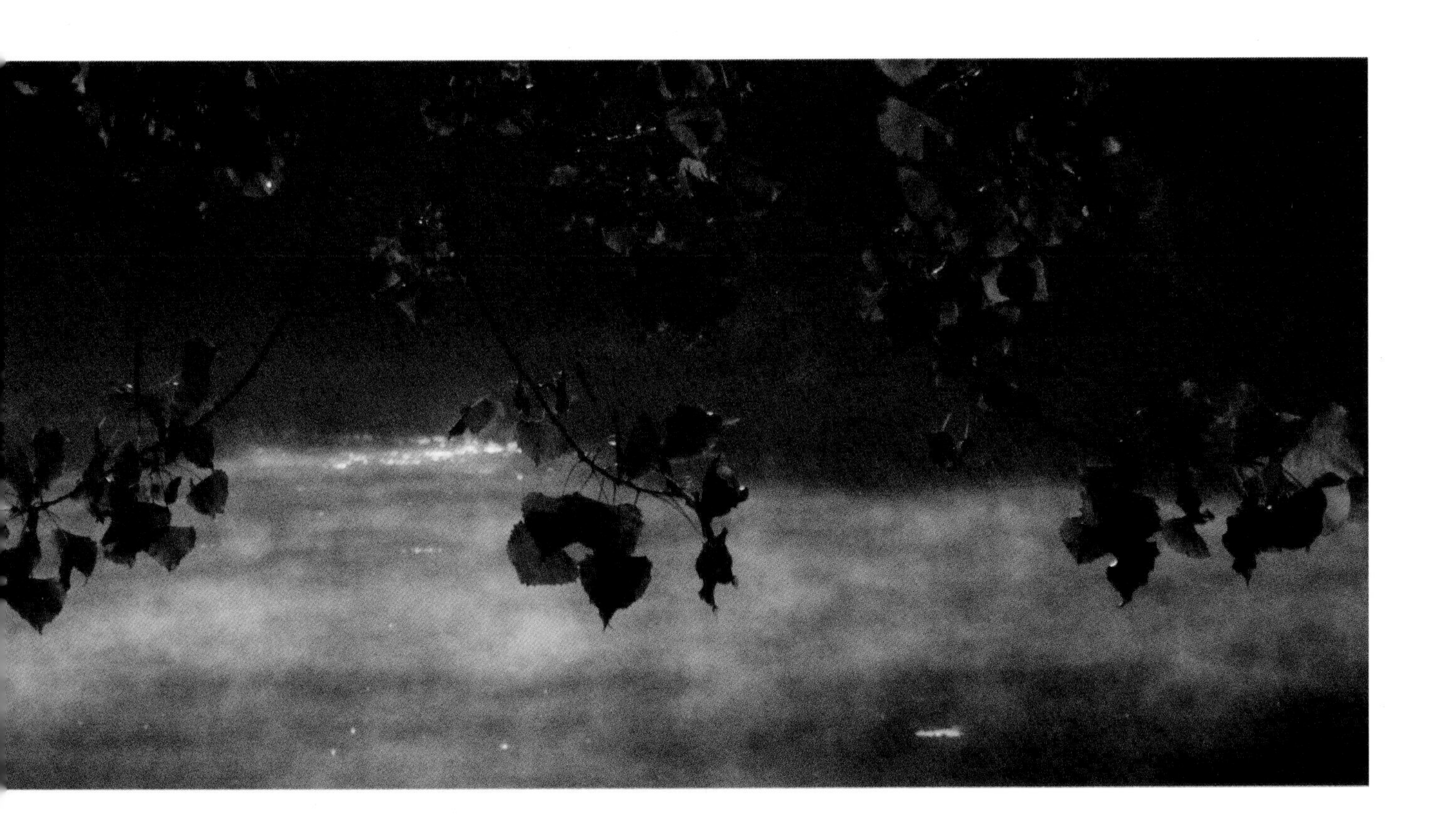

Today's rain
Will raise the lake
Another inch or so.

The dry woods
And thirsty roots
Are pulling water
Down
And
Up,
Emerging into emerald leaves,
Into catkins,
Buds,
Blossoms,
Carapaces of emerging life.

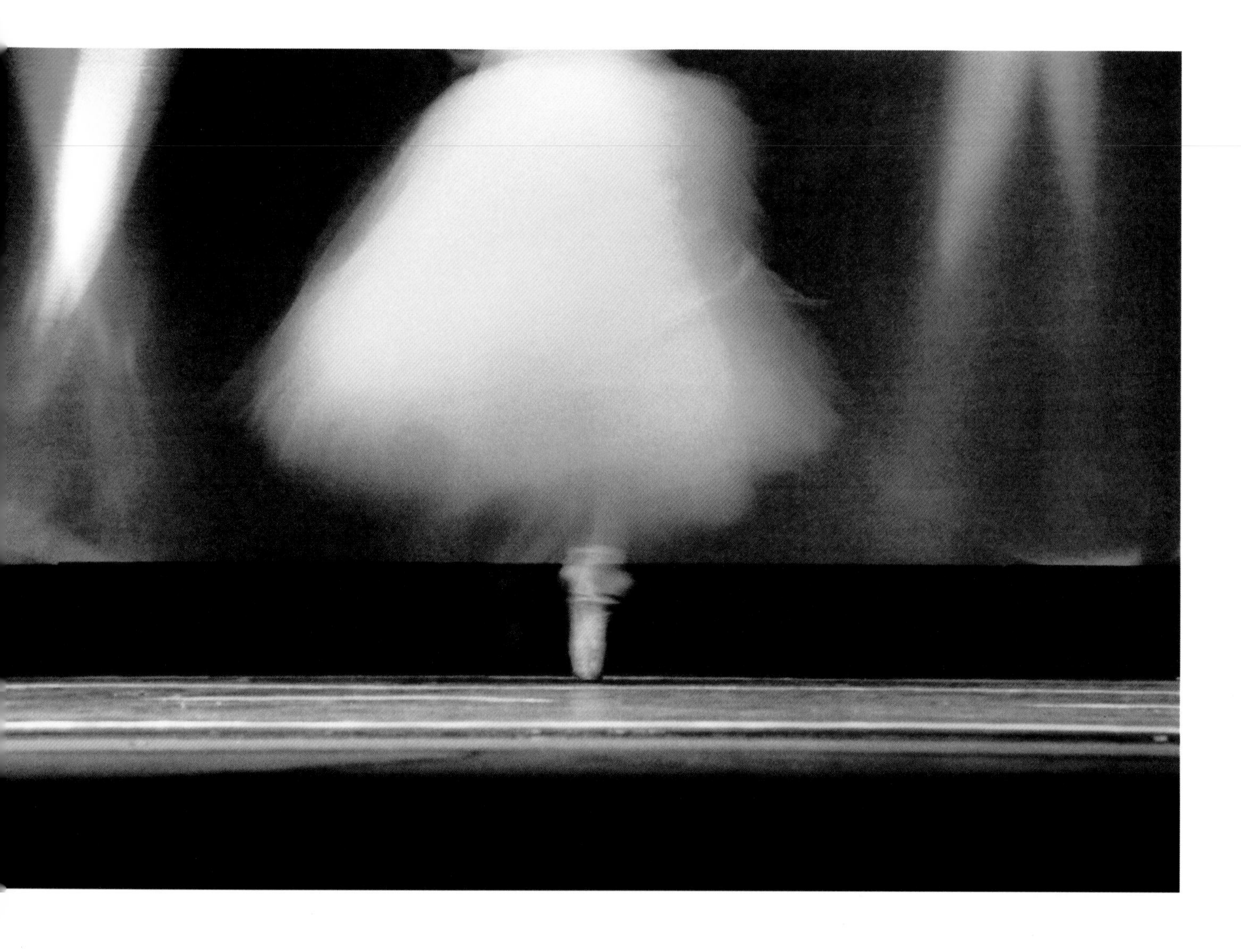

Trees,
Like mountains,
Reach up
Against gravity
To a particular point
Of instability.

What happens to me
When I grow so far
I reach
My own uncertainty?

Trees bend
And break
Altering elements of energy
Through time.

Mountains fragment,
Pushed by wind
And cracked by frost;
Breaking rocks
Slide down as scree
To balance pressures
Up and down.

Is death
The upper limit
Beyond which
Energy returns
To final
And more stable
Forms?

On Toe, Tornstrom Auditorium, Brainerd, Minnesota 1995 | 10/26/99

I walk through snow
In someone else's tracks,
And where they end,
Begin mine.

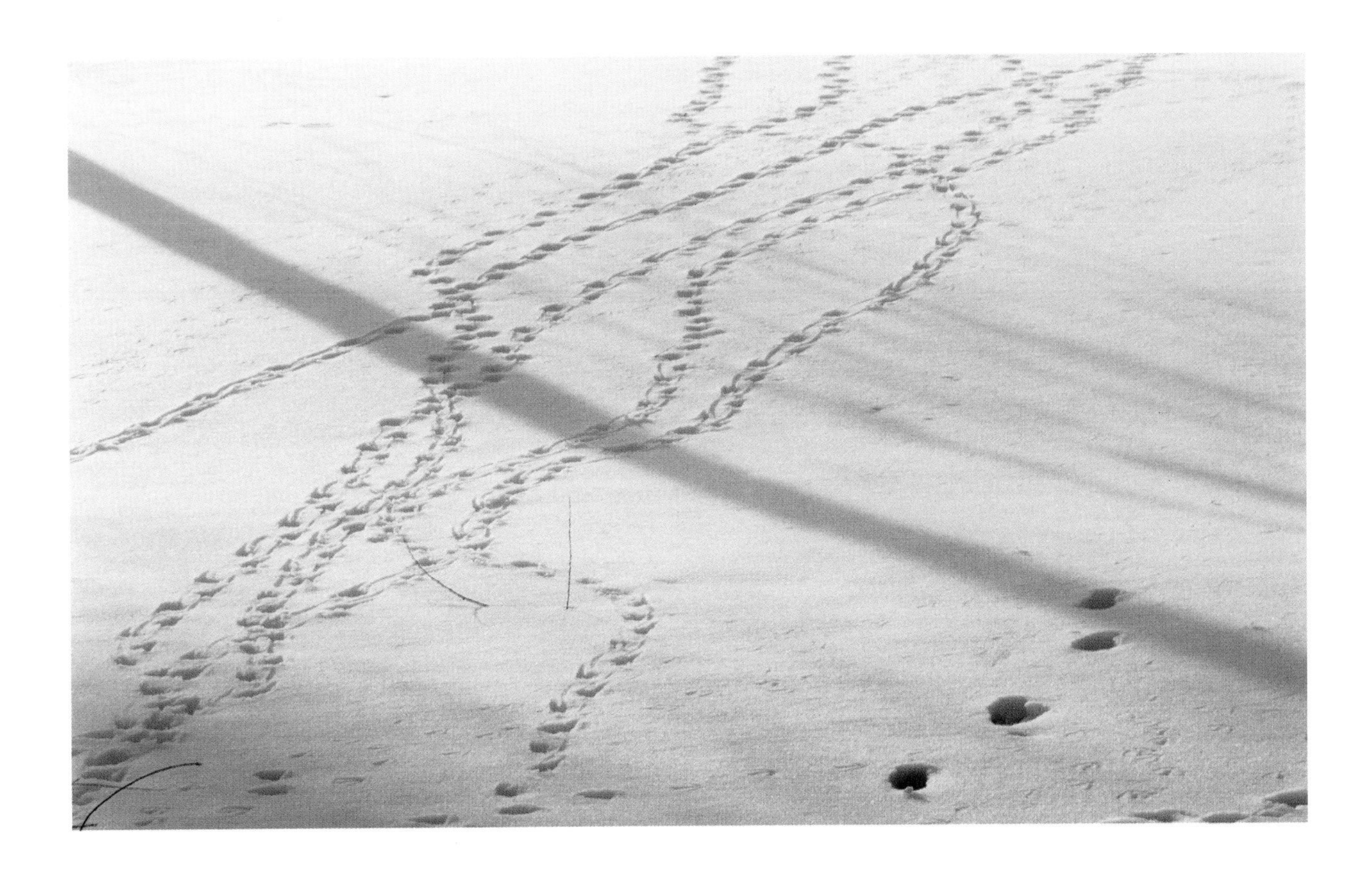

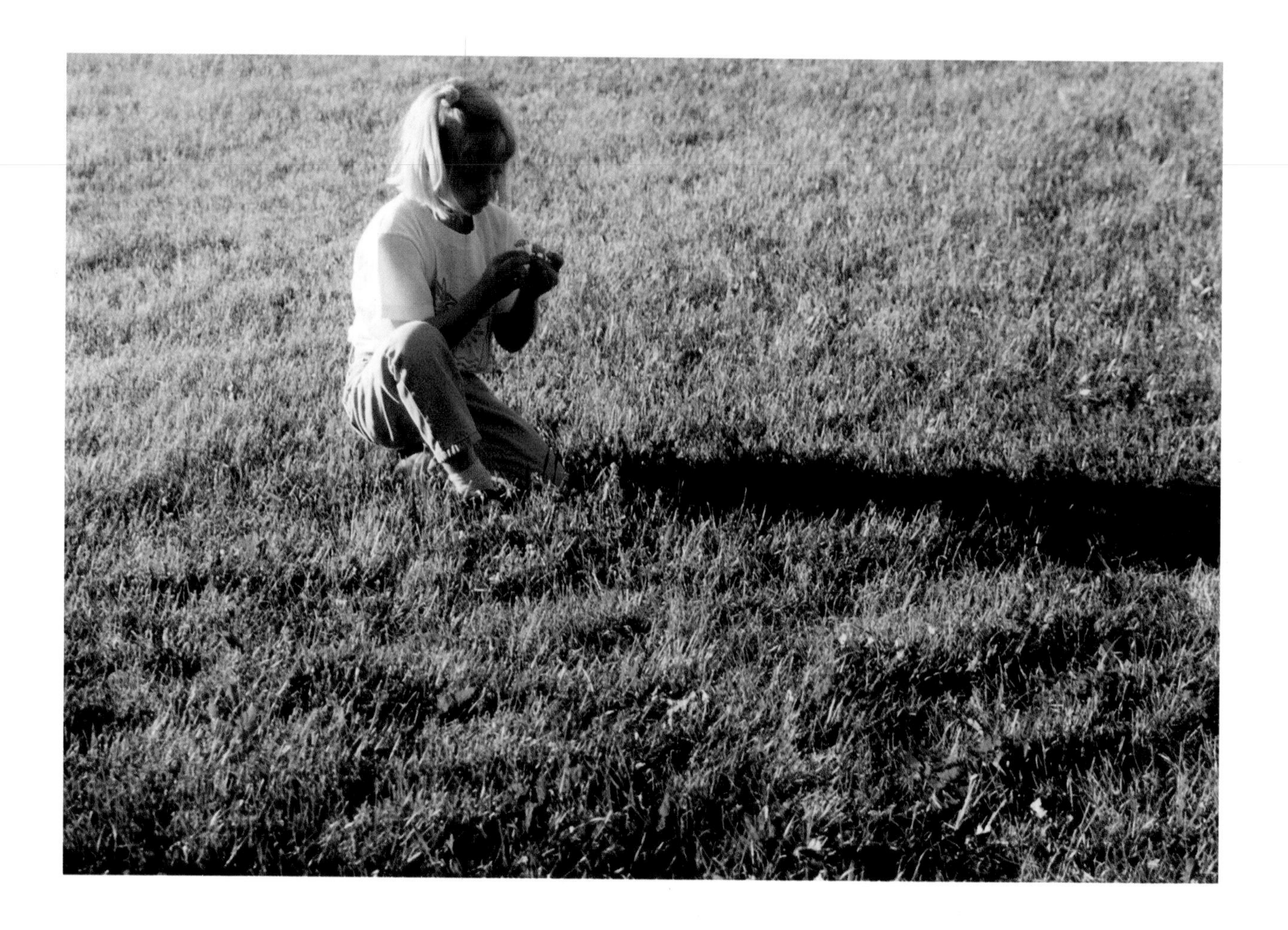

If I soften the shell
That covers my soul,
Will it hurt?
Will I die?

11/29/84

Swedish Girl, Lum Park, Brainerd, Minnesota 1997

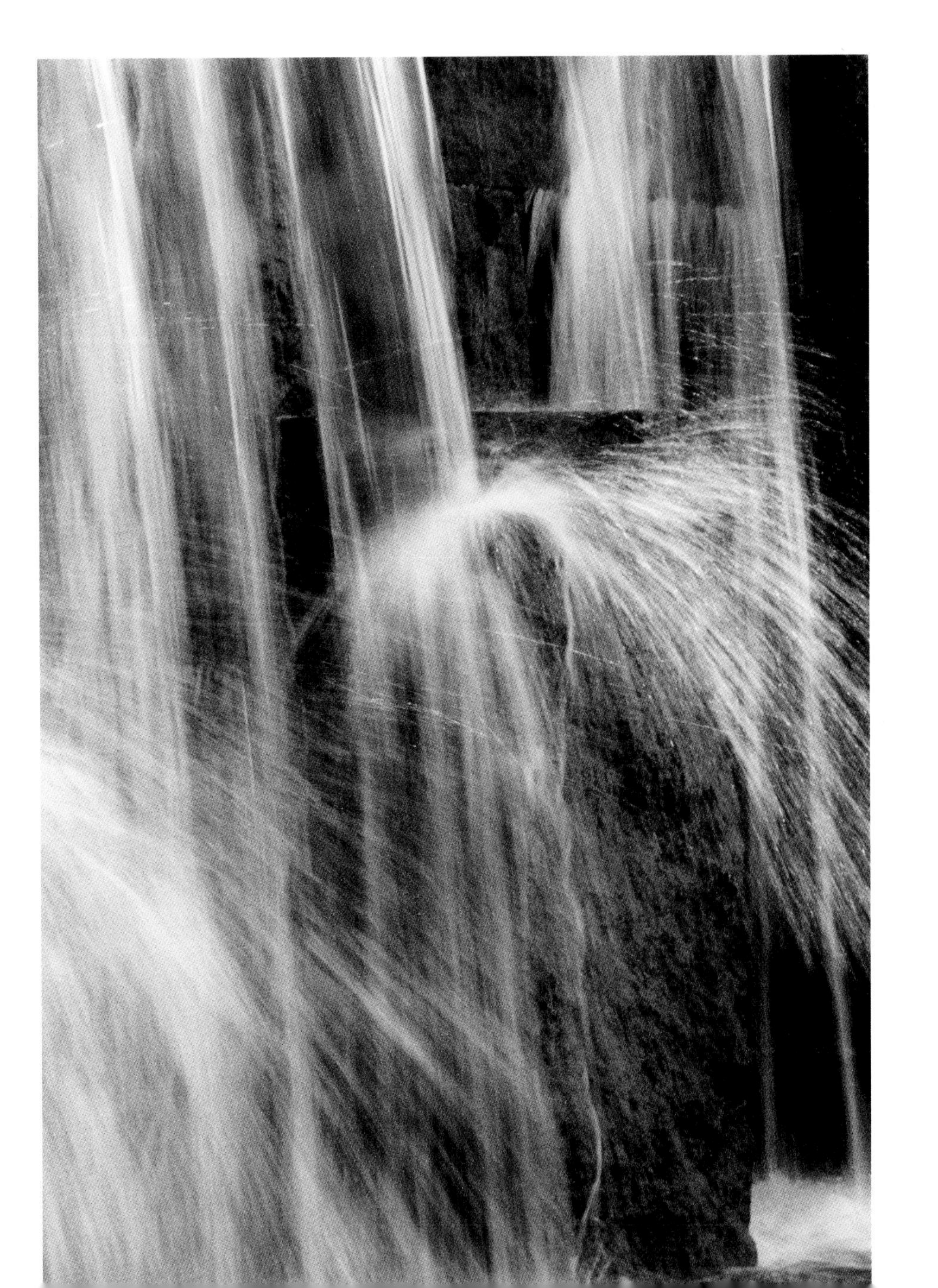

Your laughter,
Like a tiny waterfall,
Cascades in prismed rivulets
Along a widening watercourse.

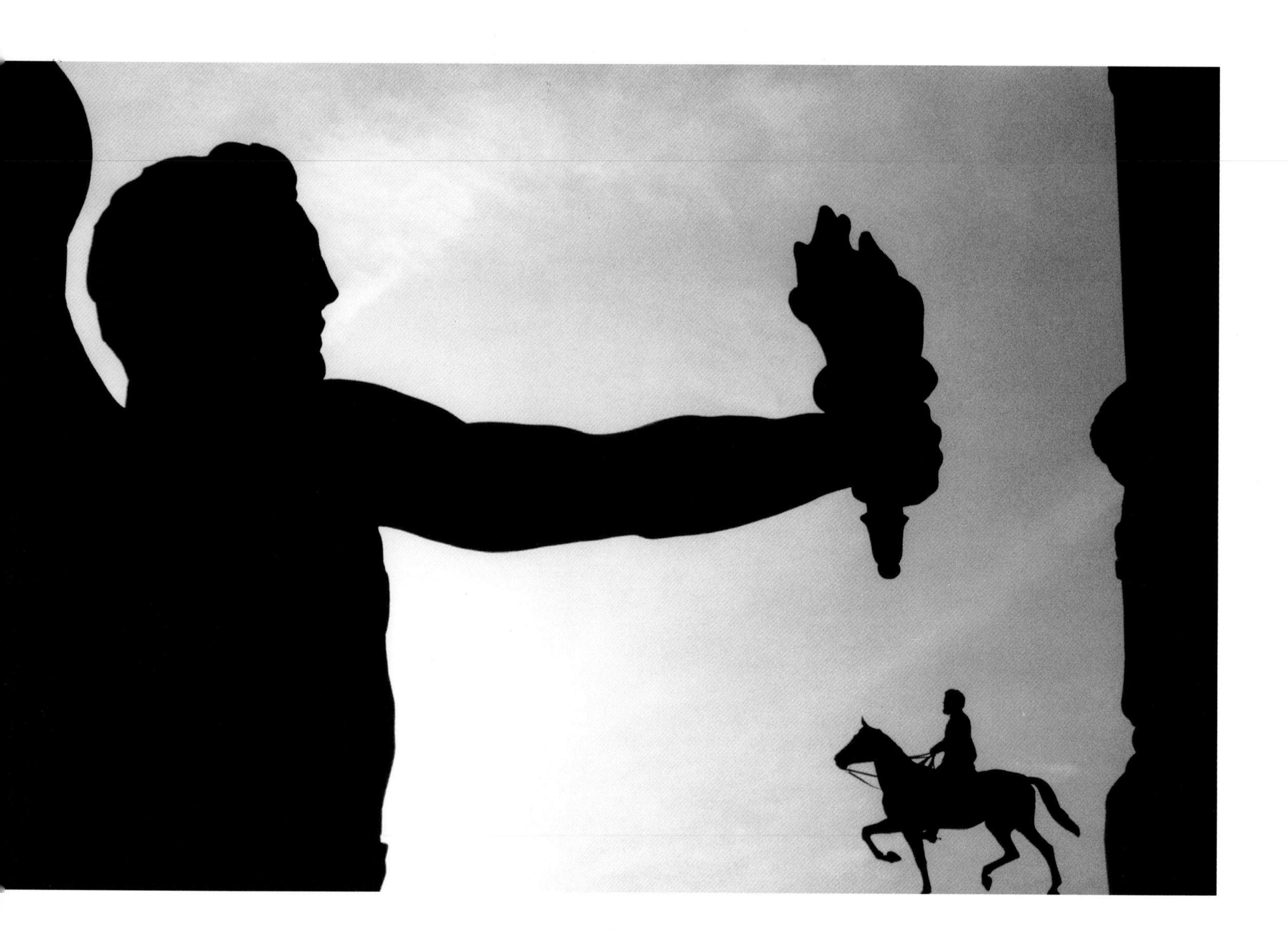

Statuary, Capitol Grounds, Des Moines, Iowa 1993 | 09/29/01

SACRIFICED TO THIS GOD:
September 11, 2001 8:45 AM EDT

Not with neck-wrung doves,
Nor throat-slit oxen,
Nor slaughtered sheep,
Was this god's indifference summoned to attention,
This god's apparent anger satisfied,
Our unacknowledged sins atoned for.

It was with the blood of children,
Women,
Men,
That this god was courted
And appeased.

"Impact airspeed: 200+ knots."

Impartial readouts of temperature,
Air pressure,
Altitude and airspeed,
GPS coordinates,
Taken together,
Established,
For an instant,
The moment this god might have intervened,
But didn't.

Gripping the control column,
Turning the wheel,
Pushing the rudder pedals,
The airborne acolyte of this god
Drove
Tons of aluminum and steel,
His body,
And all the bodies with him,
Into an unforgiving wall.

The radome,
First to arrive,
Shredded itself,
Torn by glass and stainless steel.

The unbreakable,
Heated windshields shattered.

Cockpit instruments,
All within the tolerances of their own unique accuracy,
Stopped sensing,
Abruptly,
Along with children,
Women,
Men,
Who had no choice,
No voice in this act of human sacrifice,
United forever,
In this one instant of annihilation.

Who was this god?

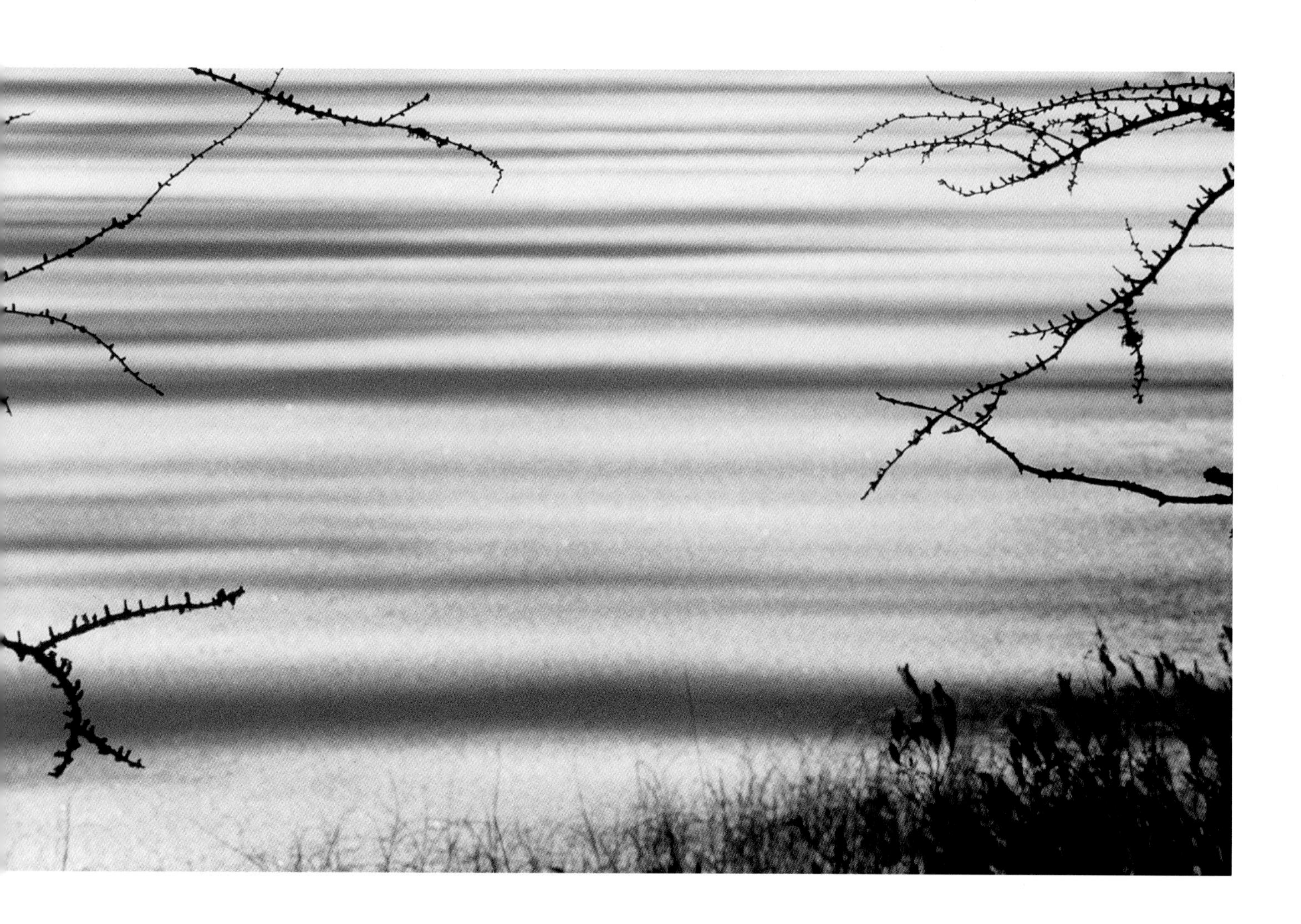

December 22nd:
The days are getting longer,
So is my life.

Forgiveness
Cannot be compromised
Without
Distorting its meaning.

A long dead lake,
Covered by flat snow
Sprouts pine trees
Here and there.

Cold snow
Drops silently,
Drifts delicately,
Making tracks
Disappear.

Pond at Winter, LaPlant's Place, Garrison, Minnesota 2001 | 12/30/96

Winter Light, Mississippi River, Brainerd, Minnesota 1997

Lake ice grumbles,
Swelling up,
Continuing to freeze
In warm Spring air.

Strong winds
Lift last night's ice
In sparkling shards;
Birdflocks of them
Cross the lake.

By the way I live,
At the edge of no thing,
I create
Every thing.

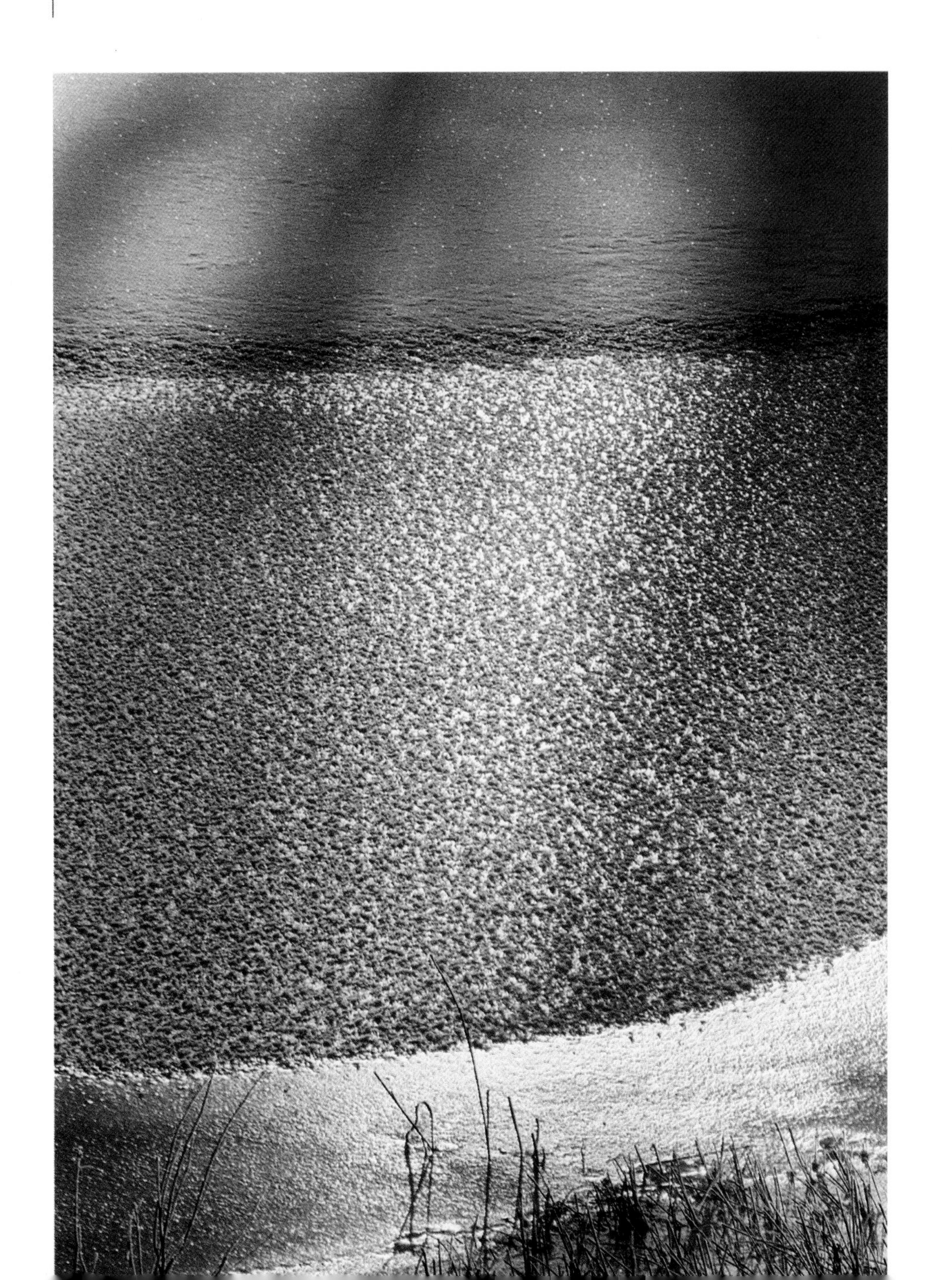

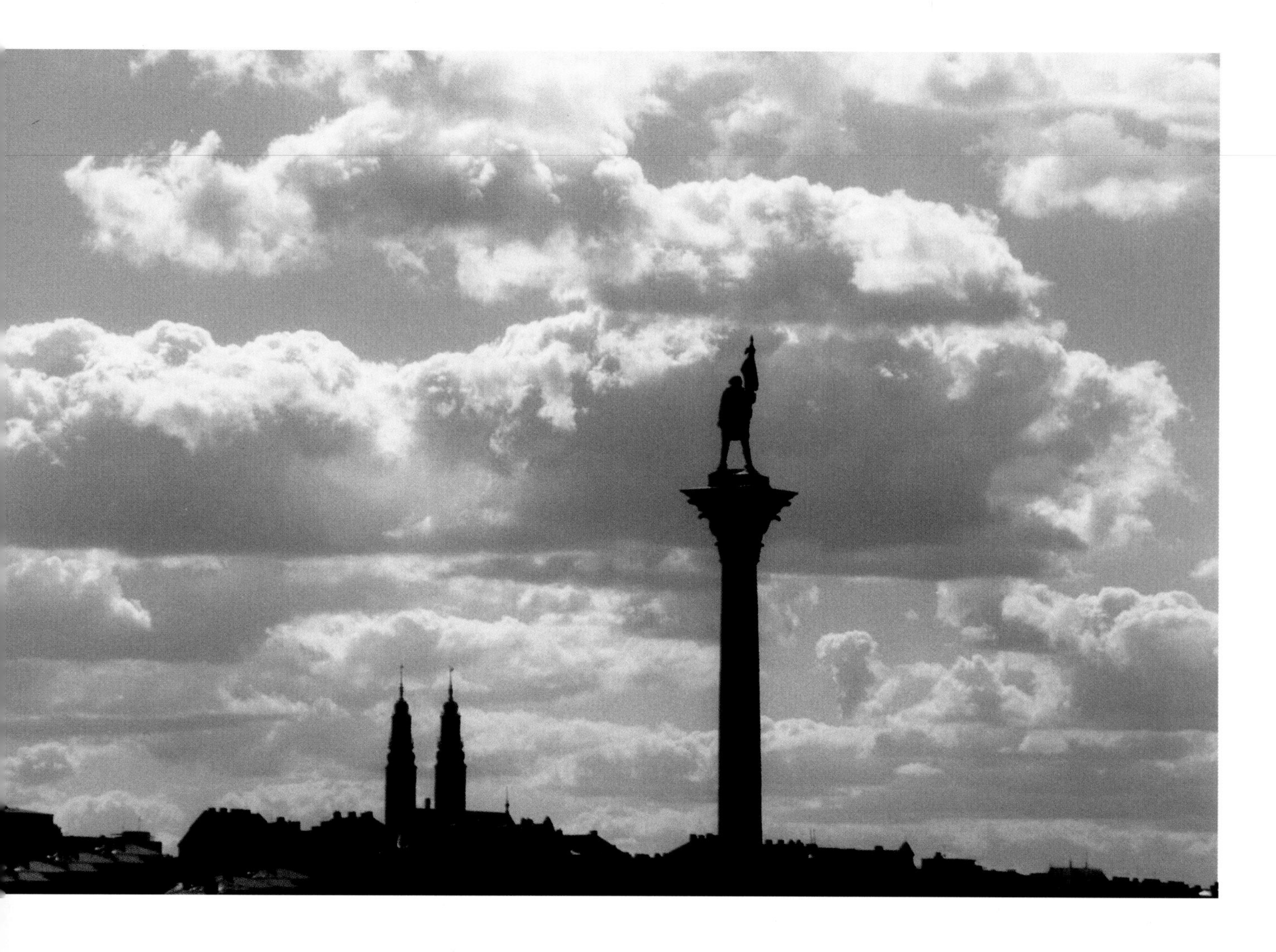

When I die
I'll be part of the sky
And live in the clouds
Forever!

Gustav Vasa, Stockholm, Sweden 1997 | 06/06/99

Silence, Flood Bay, Lake Superior, Near Two Harbors, Minnesota 1999

Between loose layers,
Sunset charges a furnace in the west
And,
In a moment,
It is gone.

Lake waves spatter lightly on the shore,
Delicate contempt spits wetness into stones,
Sliding greenness edges into deep.
Slabs of silver break up yards away.

Rounded rubble lumped in ledges lifts
Directed eyes to sharp horizons.

Shafts of heat and dark on prominences
Vomit clouds of grit and stink
That slink along the wretched rocks
And puffs of drifting poison slide across
the tension of the lake.

Echoes of a distant past writhe gasping
on the stones
And traces of one agony
Contort the brittle bones
Of flattened fishes forced by fate
To arch their gaping maws at men
As they disintegrate.

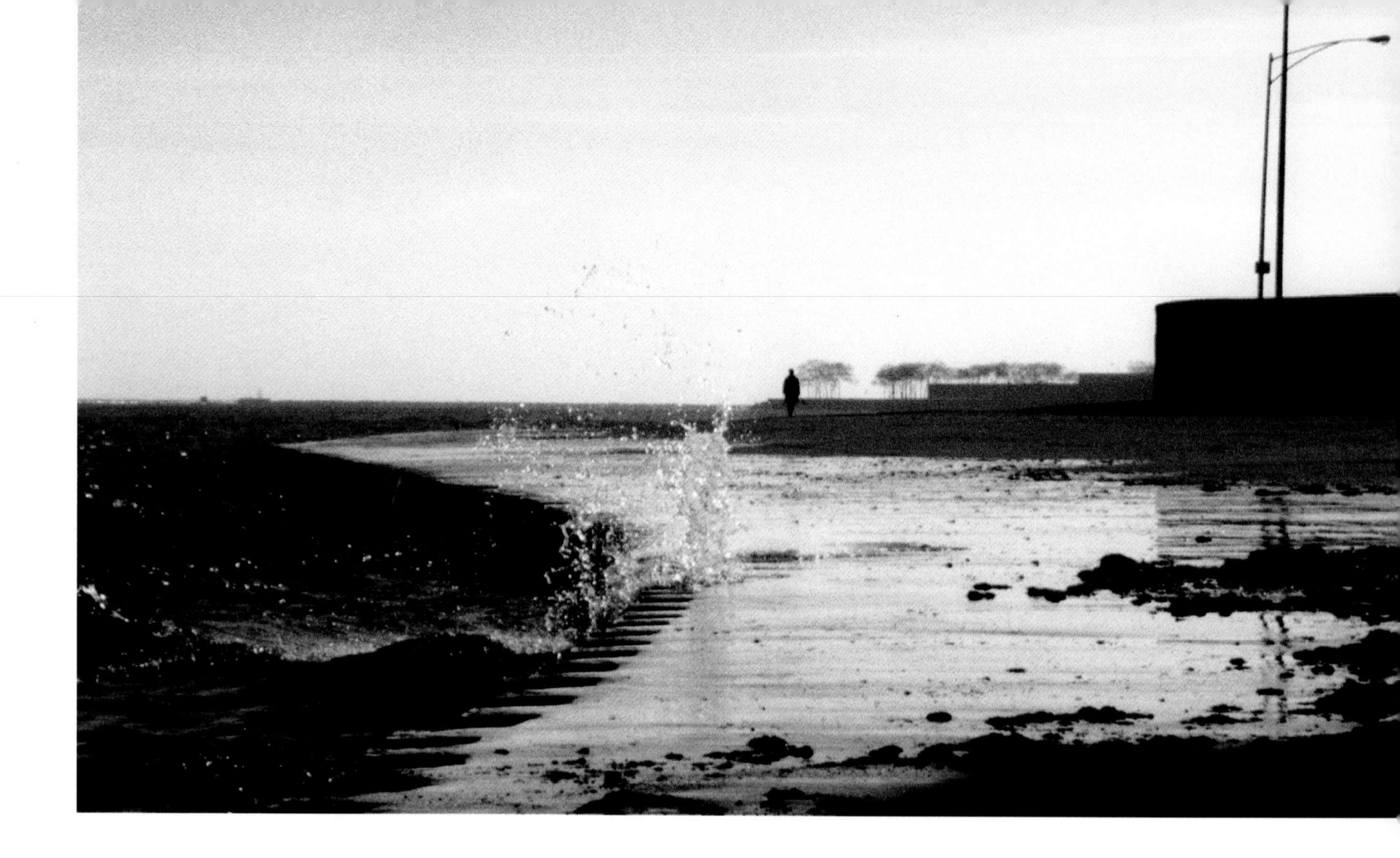

Along the stumbling backbone
hung with sand,
Evasive clumps and clusters stand erect,
Occasionally bending, searching out
the flattest slabs
To send them skipping through the air
And chatter troughs of troubled glass.

The long lake mews and waits its turn,
Covers its head and flicks its arrogance at men
Who sense the signals of the sun
And plod reluctantly to problems they had left.

06/18/63

Figure Alone on Lakewalk, Lake Michigan, Chicago, Illinois 1994

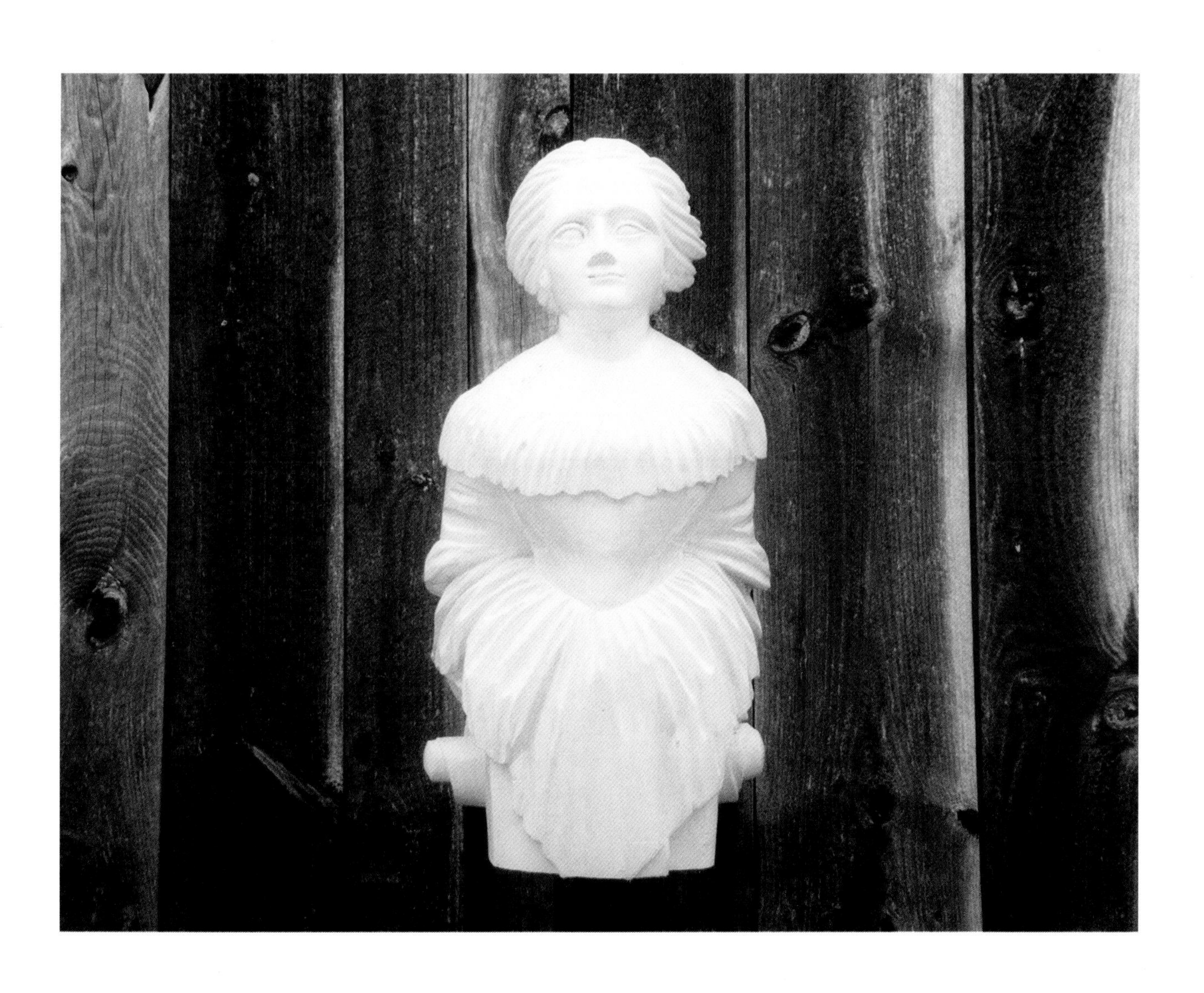

Your alert green eyes
are catching me
the way velvet marigolds are.

Oh Lord, I want to dance with you!
And you know it.
Your feet and lips and fingers show it.

I haven't danced with anyone else
Since we had our hands and heads together.

Or maybe I did—but I really didn't;
Apart from you, I can't—and I couldn't.

I hated to hear that wall-to-wall waltz,
To feel you so close
And your laughter beside . . .

How quickly we ran up the fantasy tree
When you were just you
And I was just me!

Ainsi soit-il!

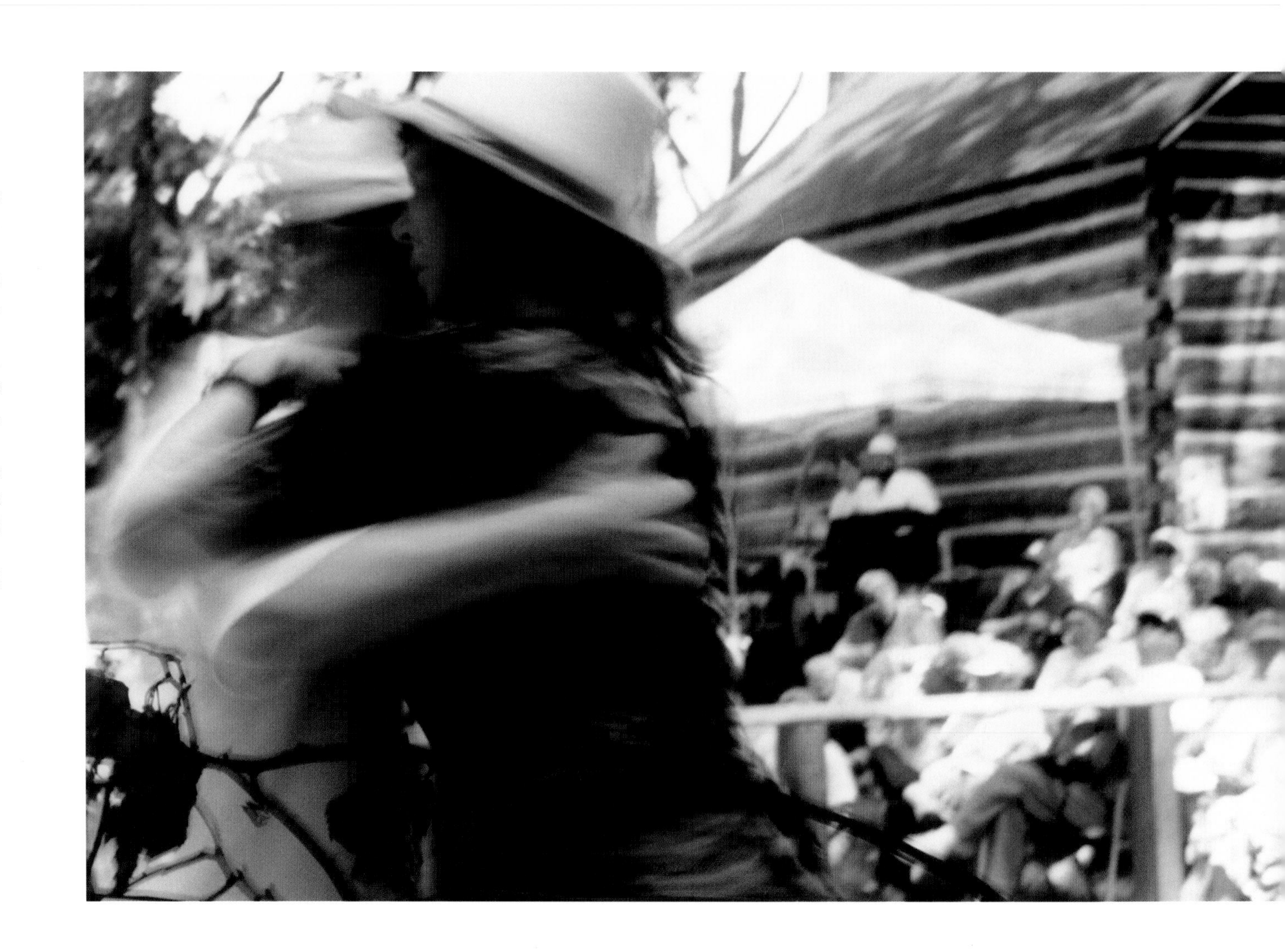

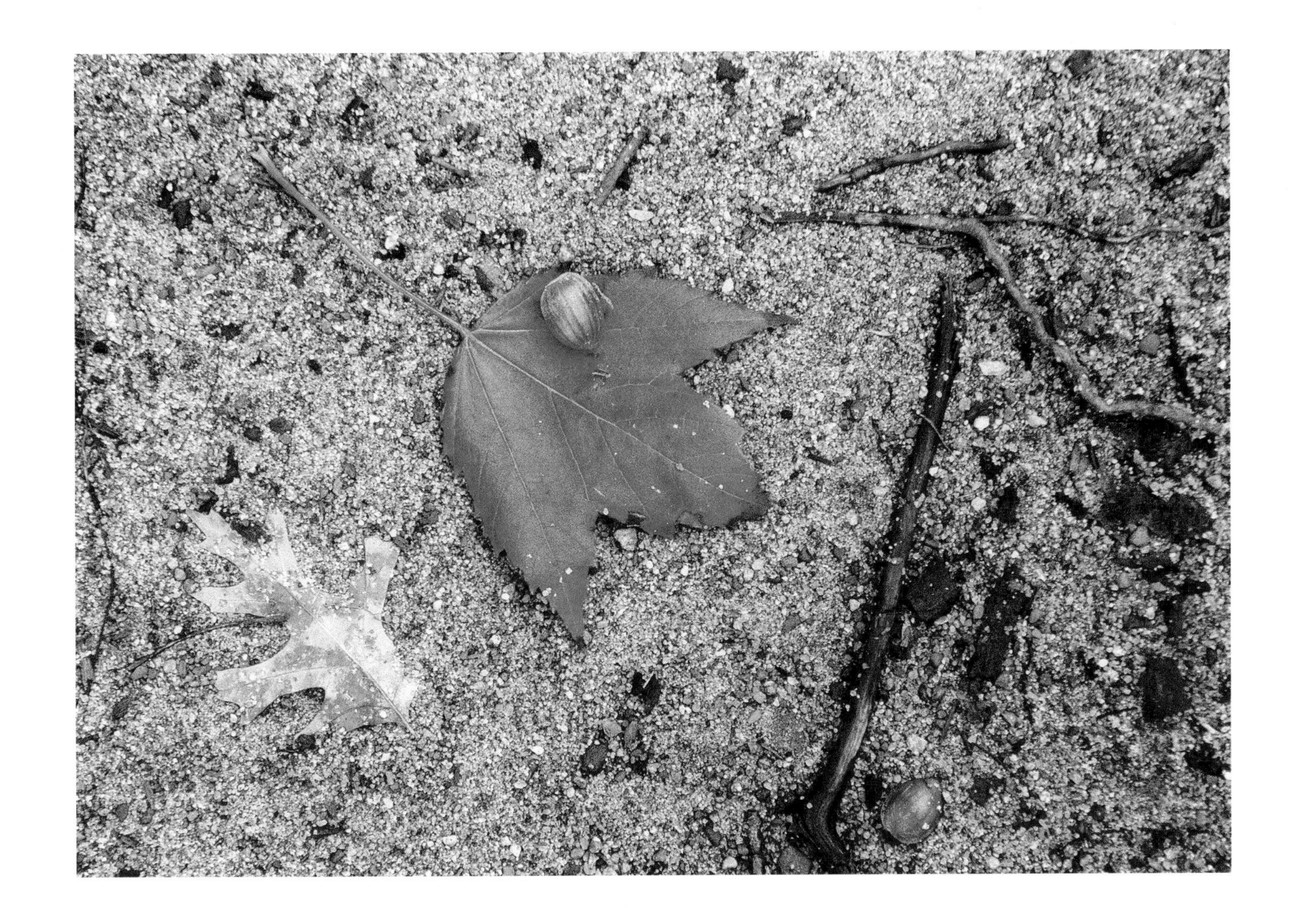

An acorn falling in the night
Strips a slender cylinder of sound
Brushing breaking branching buds
Before impact.

Beginning, End, Riverton, Minnesota 1997 | 07/08/71

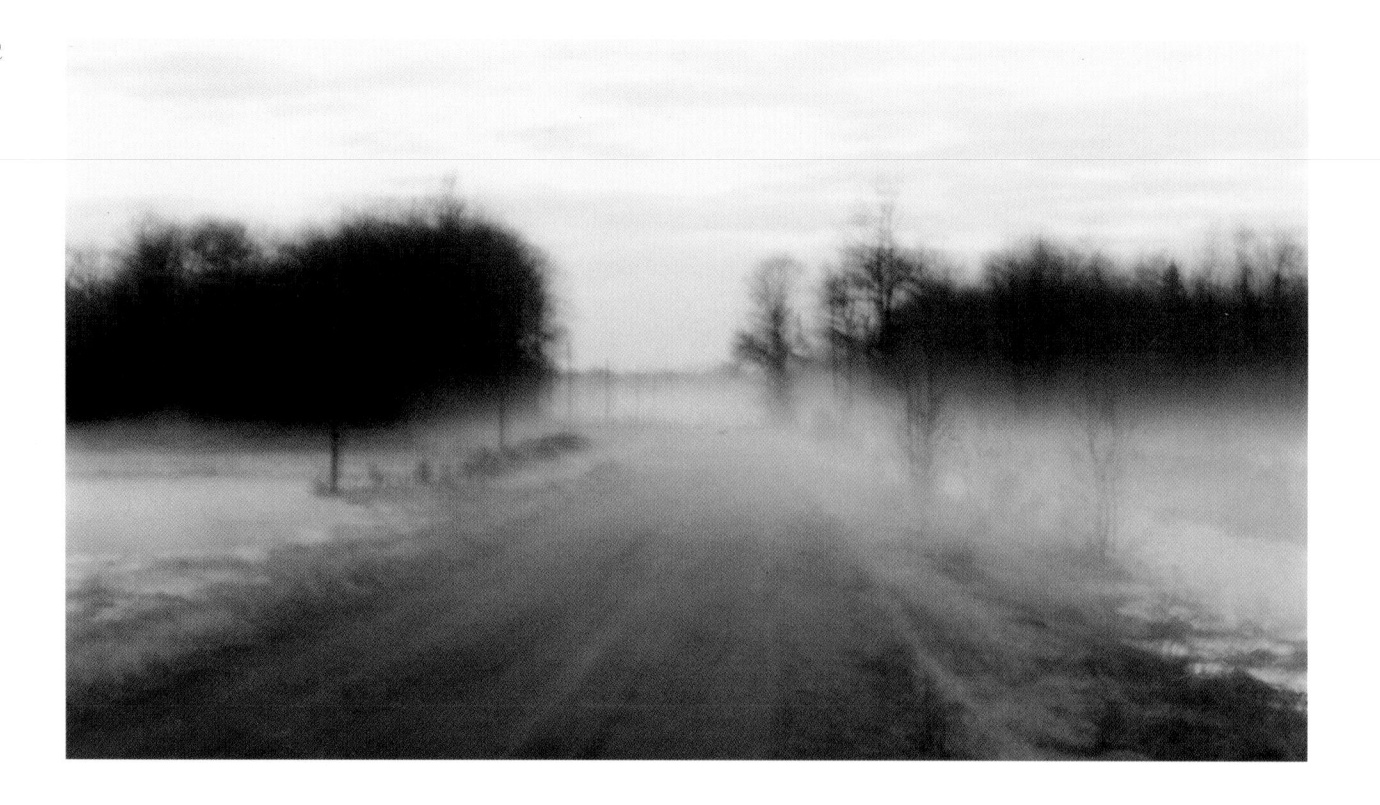

Warm air
Edges slowly,
Through the woods,
Over the burden
Of last year's snow.

Settling softly,
Warm air disappears
Into ground cloud.

There is no other place
To go.

Exit from 210, Aitkin County, Minnesota 1995 | 03/31/97

Where will I awake,
And be me?

Am I the dreaming dreamer,
Imagining a world,
Imagining a world?

How can I separate
The "might be"
From the "what is"?

Am I not the awkward mixture
Of my stepping forward,
Holding back?

The really real
Presents itself in pain,
A postponed parturition
Birthing new meanings
Breathlessly,
And unaware.

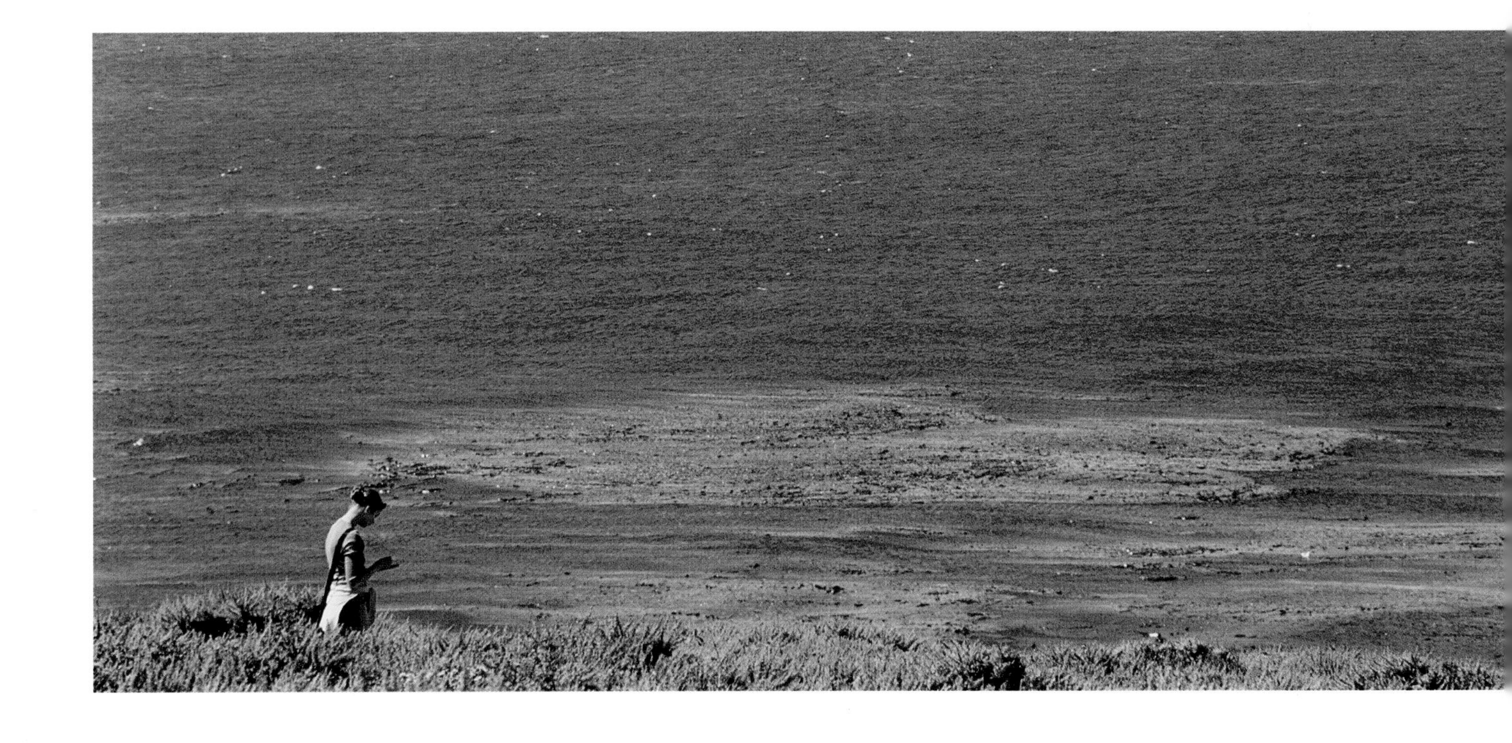

Stand with me
By the shag-bark hickory.
The grass here and there
Suppressed by weathered slabs
Torn off by wind
Or fingered out by frost.

Roll back your head
And trace with me
The edges of impulsive filigree
Etched against the blotter grey
Of today's sky.

Her leaves are gone;
Her children,
Dropped and weathered,
Point careful lines
In all directions.
None seem to notice her
Or care.

For her great strength exists
To lift them up
In seminality,
To offer opportunity
For vision
And unhindered growth.

For her own life
A cup of earth
Will someday be too much;
When some strong storm
Begins to break
The rigid reaches
Of her arms;

When all the jealous hosts
Begin to bore
The riches of her form;
When no Spring rain
Or Summer sun
Replaces the will
To die.

I do not wish to see her down
And dead,
But ask that you
Make here
With me

A celebration
Or creation
In this tree
With me.

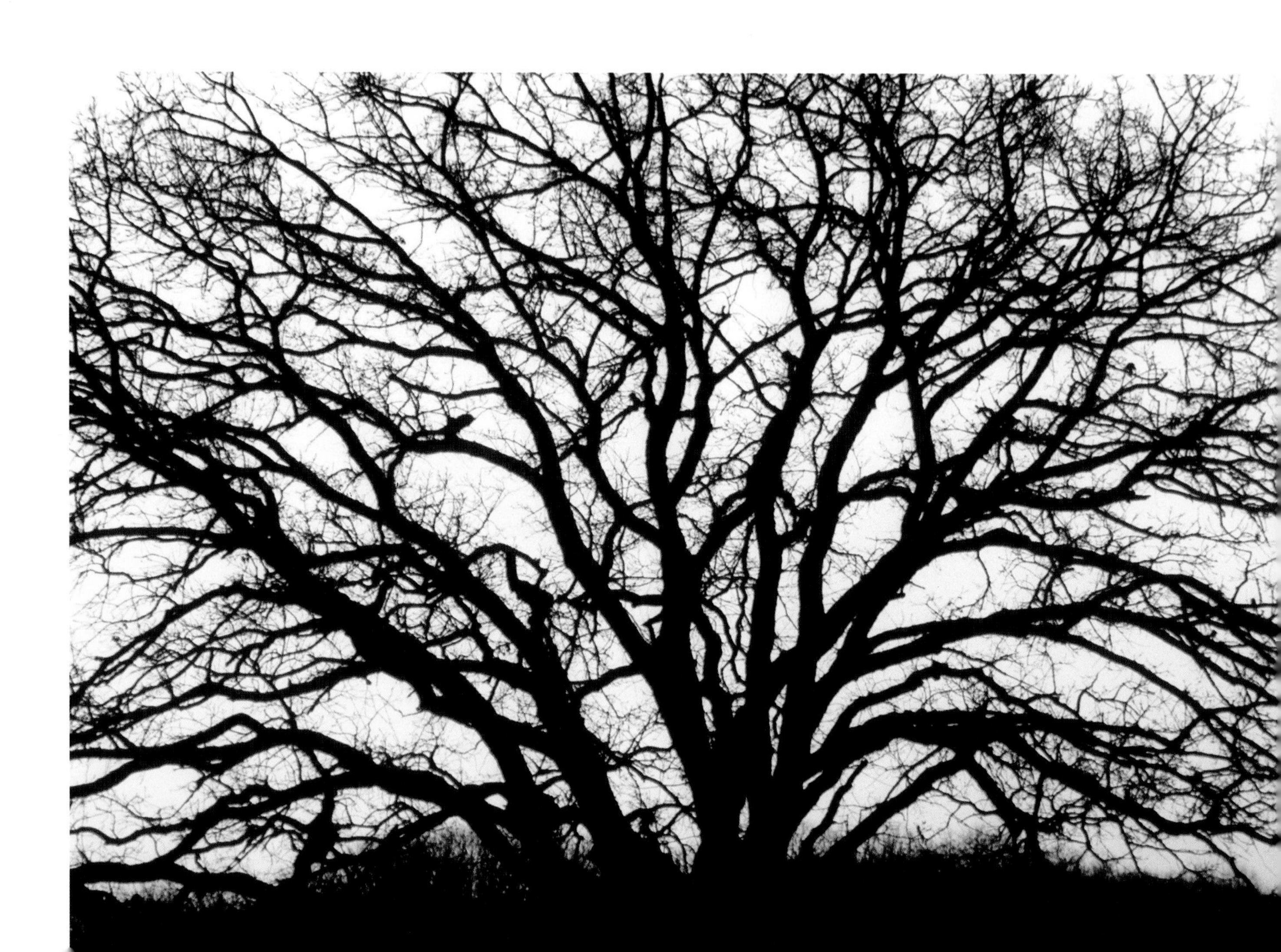

The shag-bark hickory:

Today I'm tracing memories,
The signs of having been there,
Then.

The shag-bark hickory is gone!
No trace remains.
Concrete slabs
Are scabs
Covering the open sore
Where she once stood,
Where roots ran deep,
Where life coursed up,
And through,
And out those outstretched arms
That blossomed
And bore fruit.

Did that tree die of grief,
Or with relief
That Winter storms
And Summer sun
No longer try to bend
Or break
The impulse at her heart?

I wanted to see it one more time.
I wanted to remember you
Again.

I wanted you.
I wanted you to stand with me
Beside the shag-bark hickory.

I wanted you to hear me say,
"I love you!"

I wanted you to know
How much my heart hurt
To say,
"Goodbye!"
To turn away,
Alone.

Through my stifled tears
I spoke to that tree,

Invoking you beside me.
The tree was a crossing place,
A reaching out to you across the barriers
Of space
And time.

What if the tree is gone?
It was.
There.
It is,
Now,
In my words
To you.

The tree's decay
Is her way
Of feeding life
Again,
Unseen,
In silence.

You are with me
Beside that tree
In more than memory.

We are,
And always will be together
In that tree
Continuing creation.

09/17/01

Alone,
Against a darkling sky,
Absence of leaves
Reveals the delicate tracery
Of branches impelled outward
By the orderly impulses
Of life,
Itself.

Life At Dawn, Near Faribault, Minnesota 1997 | 10/29/01

Reflected Branch at Dawn, December Water, Lakeville, Minnesota 1998

Stillness
Creates the opportunity
For symmetry.

Is the world symmetrical
Or not?

Does this reflection tell us
Anything
About what reality
Really is?

Sometimes
I think I take the reflection
Itself
To be the thing
Itself.

How can a world,
A universe,
A multiverse,
Exist
Where both
Are possible?

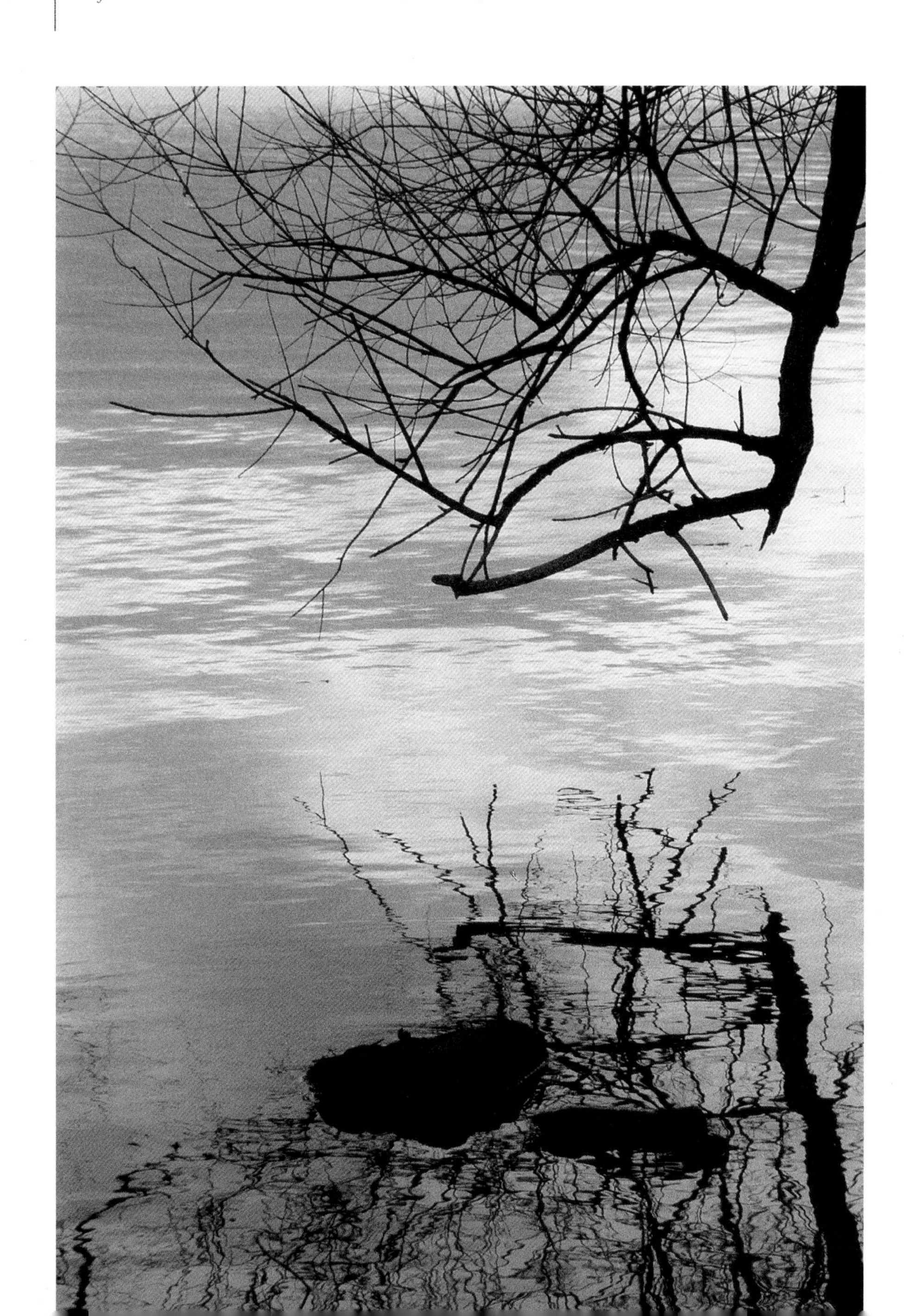

Sunlight thins in September,
Sliding sideways
Across dusty,
Drying fields
And trees.

Even the air is hesitant,
Holding softness,
Warmth,
And strength;
Holding against sadness,
Tears and emptiness;
Holding for a moment
All there is in me;

Remembering in memory,
Imagining in fantasy,
Being there,
In reality.

Field at Dawn, Fall, Near New Prague, Minnesota 1998 | 09/28/58

Distant Sky, December Dawn, Lakeville, Minnesota 1998

Seven miles,
Seven miles high,
A hundred miles away,
Flying into the settling sun,
Straining to see into the
deepening darkness,
Knowing where people and
places should be,
Not being able to resolve them in
the growing gloom,
Or in my past,
Or in my present,
But there they are,
Over there,
Away in the slowly sliding silence.

I want to see them clearly,
But I can't—
So much always depends on
approximations
And imaginings.

I can barely see my own reflection
In the cracked and crazed plastic window.

Around the yellowed edges of a
minor rainbow,
Light broken into bits,
They frame my musings,
Reassembled in a ring.

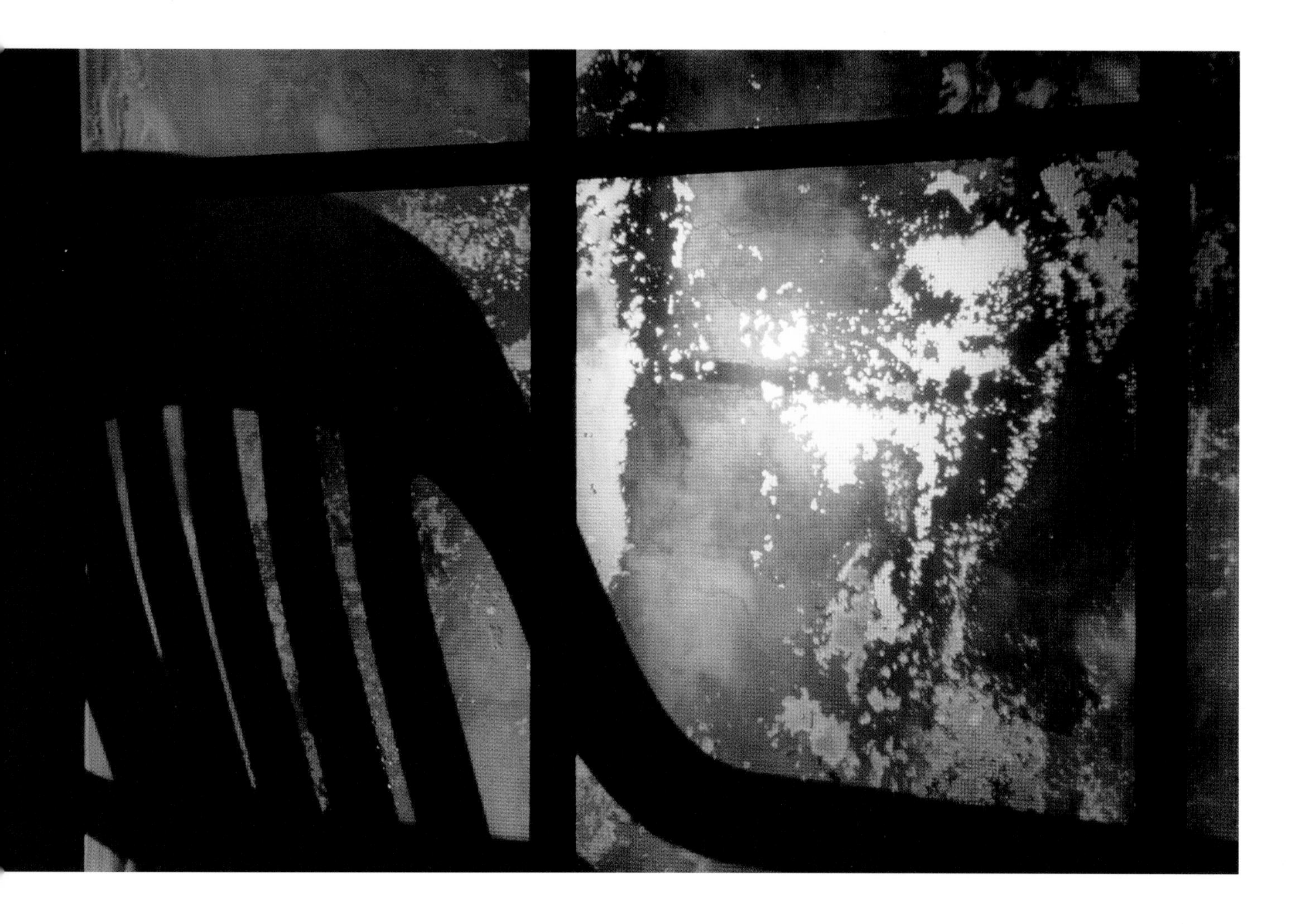

It took an hour
To empty her room
The day after she died.

Bags and boxes
Held everything left of her life.

Not much to do:
A closet full of dresses
Going to other residents
Who will wear them well.

The furniture
Was spoken for
A long time ago.
Givers got what they gave,
And more.

Small surprises,
Like earrings
And necklaces,
For those who do not know
That they are beneficiaries.

A dozen deep red roses,
Barely budding,
Stubbornly refuse to bloom
In her room.
They end up above the sink
In a dim kitchen.

A Bible,
A Christmas gift,
Probably unread
From the looks of it,
But well used,
From the looks of it;
A filing cabinet of sorts,
Obituaries,
Memories,
Reflecting fragments of lives
When they ended,
Where,
There.

Keys
And locks
And purses;
Luggage that will go
Somewhere,
Again.

Vases,
Empty.

Candy,
Scrambled
Into flat dishes,
Picked over,
Untouched.

Photographs
In frames,
In piles,
In albums,
Annotated,
Going back
Into their original images.

It took an hour,
More or less.

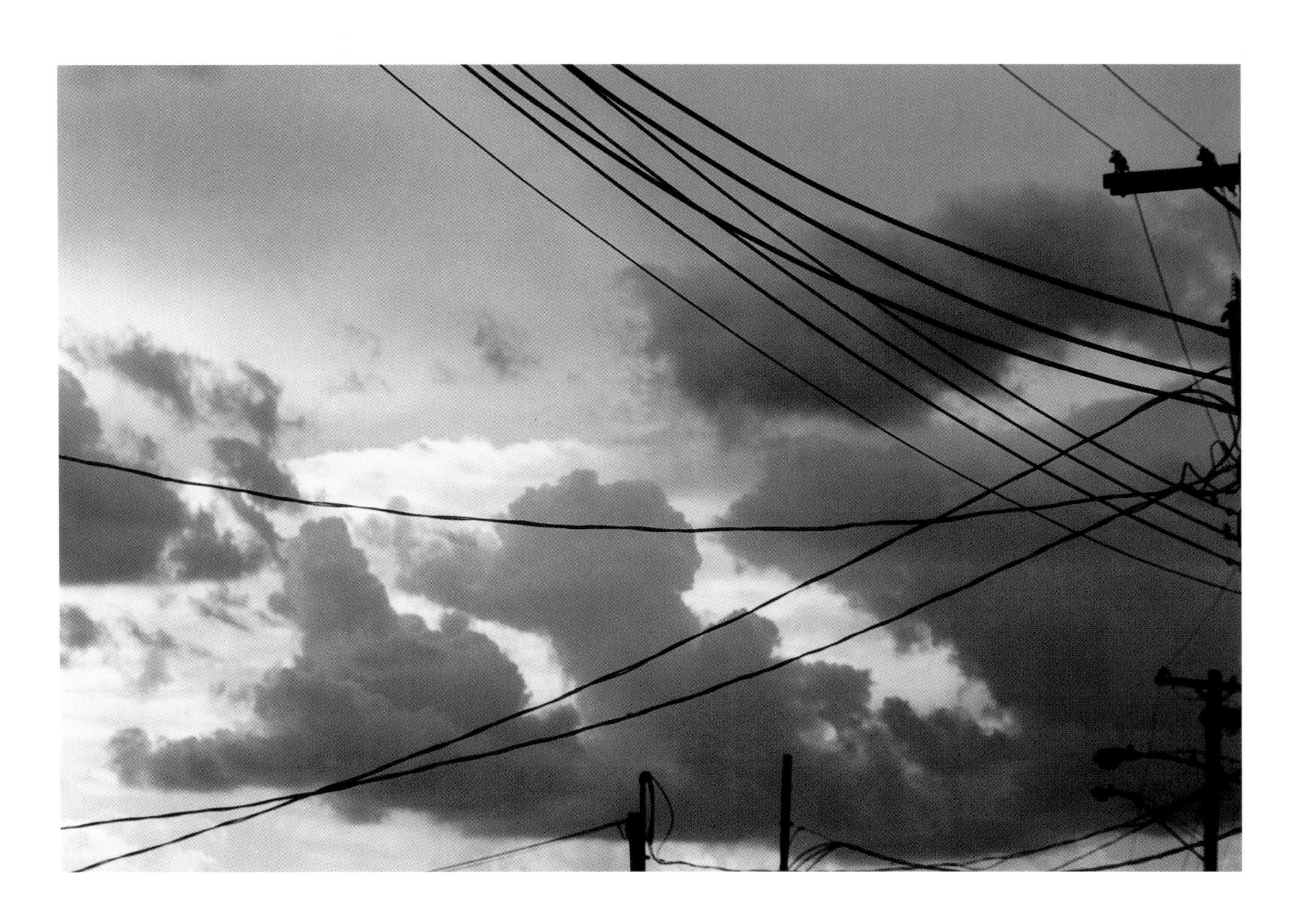

It is not always clear
How things coinhere:
Maybe they don't.
I fear.

Shadows of snowflakes,
Like swarming bees,
Build and fall
In precious patterns,
Seeking entrance,
Finding none,
They drop silently,
Together,
In one,
Delightful,
Motion.

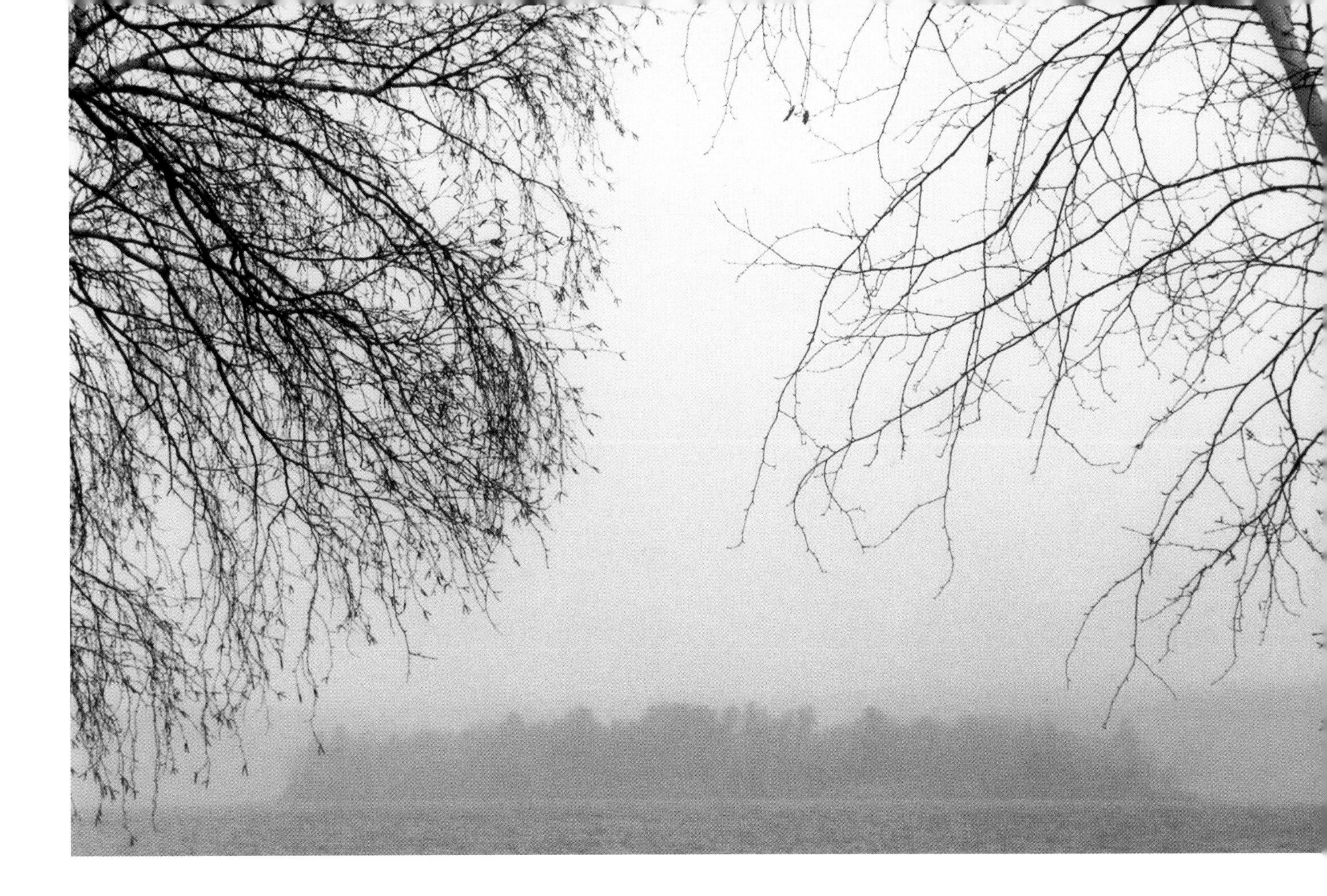

02/23/67

November, Wilson Bay, Gull Lake, Minnesota 1999

The bitter yellow moon stopped,
tauntingly,
above the trees,
daring me to find the clean white light
I crave,
Before that final shifting movement
when my backbone bends
one final time
to fit the contours of the grave.

The black sky shaped a mockery of day;
more than the absence of light and sight
I felt the lack of love and life.

There was no rest,
nor a reprieve from
all the useless loneliness,
that torment when I cried no tears
and eyesight echoed emptiness again.

Moon Risen, Lakeville, Minnesota 1998

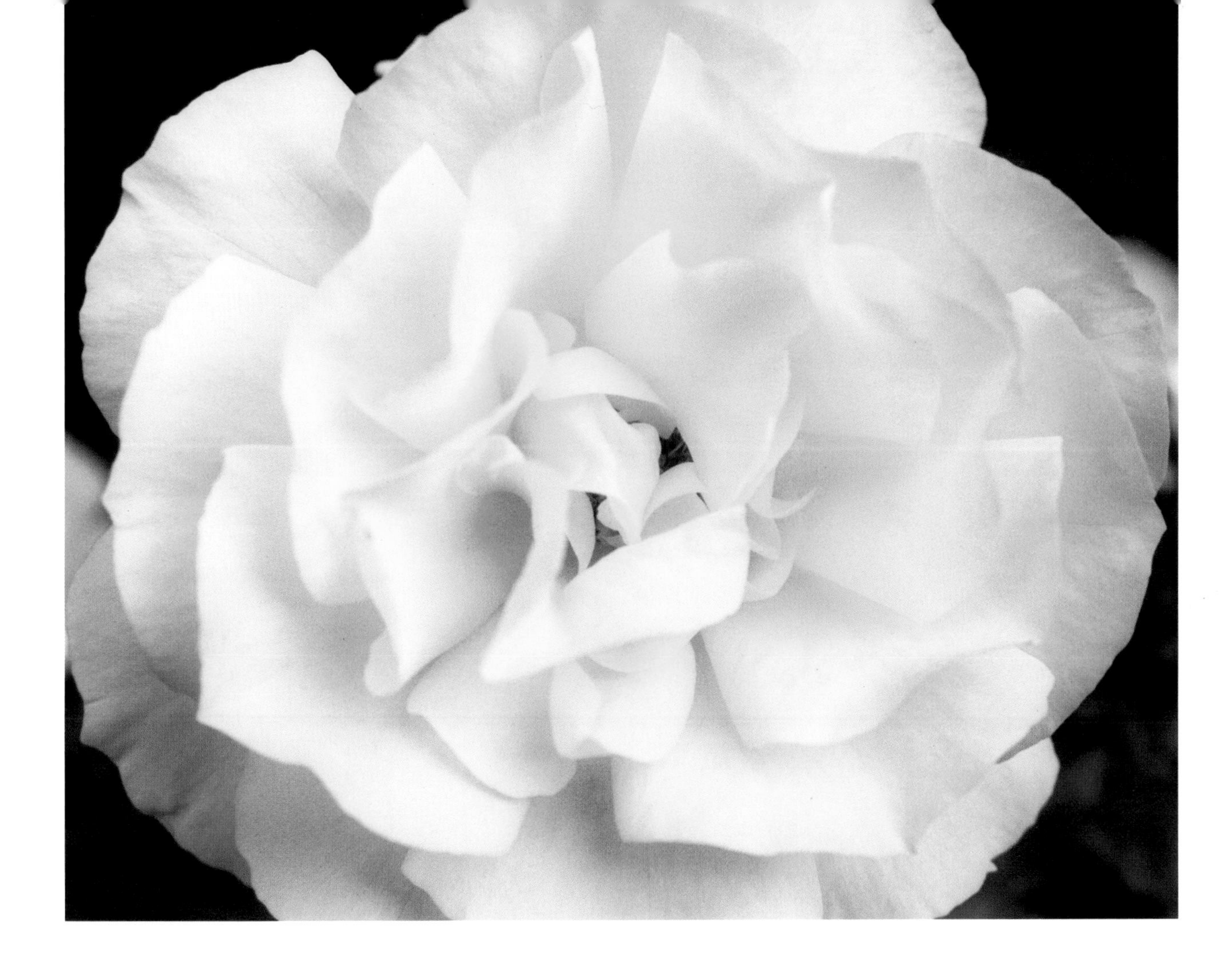

All that is,
Or ever will be,
Is present,
Now,
Here,
In this flower.

Like an old dream,
Two white roses
Bloom on one stem,
There,
In the warm dark.

Presence, Clemens-Munsinger Gardens, St. Cloud, Minnesota 2000 | 07/21/90 | 03/20/99

When you look
At me,
What do you see?
What do you really see?
Do you see me?
Or simply what you want to see
Of me?
Or are they parts of you
That you disown
And are content to see
In me?

When you really look at me,
What do you see?
Do you see the "emergency gall bladder" in room 503?
Or can you look beyond the expressions of your skill
And the inconveniences
Of looking after me
To see
The really me?

Can you detect the shades and shadows of my infant self,
The forms I filled as I grew up,
Black and unwanted,
In a hot city?
The joy and fear I felt
When I received recognition,
Stripes and service medals,
The sadness I felt
When I returned to civilian life?

Can you detect the pride I feel
In having a full family,
In seeing my children's children
Find their way
Into "Grandpa's room"
For a few unguarded moments?
Can you imagine the relief and apprehension
That I felt in coming here,
Not knowing what would happen to me,
Really?

When you look at me,
What do you see,
Really?
Do you see an old and awkward alcoholic,
Full of caries,
Poor dentition,
Suffering from malnutrition,
Unwilling to stop smoking,
Even though,
I know
That I am killing
My self?

Or can you look beyond the way that I appear,
My polyester pants
And stained shirt
To the young sailor who snapped smartly to attention
On the deck I holystoned myself?

Can you see me learning to stay
In my gun tub
In spite of nearly dying in the sun,
Sitting on the stinging seat,
Too busy to be terrified,
With burning eyes
And blistered hands,
Dropping in one clip after another,
Aiming fast fire
At the propeller
Swinging scythe-like,
Roaring toward me,
Not knowing if,
In the next few seconds,
It would slice my life,
Shred my possibilities,
Or blast and burn me
Out of my existence?

After the attack is over,
Can you hear the quietness
Of deep Pacific waters;
My bewilderment that it is all over,
For now?

Can you be still beside me as I recollect,
Or will I be just another sad statistic,
"Scut work,"
A "final four" on an MMPI,
A completed assessment
Of an uncompleted life?

When you look at me,
What do you really see?

Do you see me shuffling quietly,
Knowing my name,
But nothing else?

You take care of me;
But who am I,
To you?
Am I another "sad case,"
A patient
For whom no one at home has patience
Or endurance for the pain
Of waiting for me
To die?

Can you go back with me to my fast trip across France,
Can you join with me in my tank,
Bucking down tree-lined routes,
Across *carrefours* without slowing down
Until an 88 opened up on us
And opened us up
Flaming,
Screaming?

Can you sense the mercy
Of not remembering
My pain
Any more?

I could not,
And would not,
Share what burned into my brain that day.
The keloid scarring on my arms and legs
Reminded me
Every day
What others never had to see
In me.

My family guessed,
As best they could,
What I went through
For them
And you.

I could not speak,
And cannot now.

When you try to look at me,
What do you see?

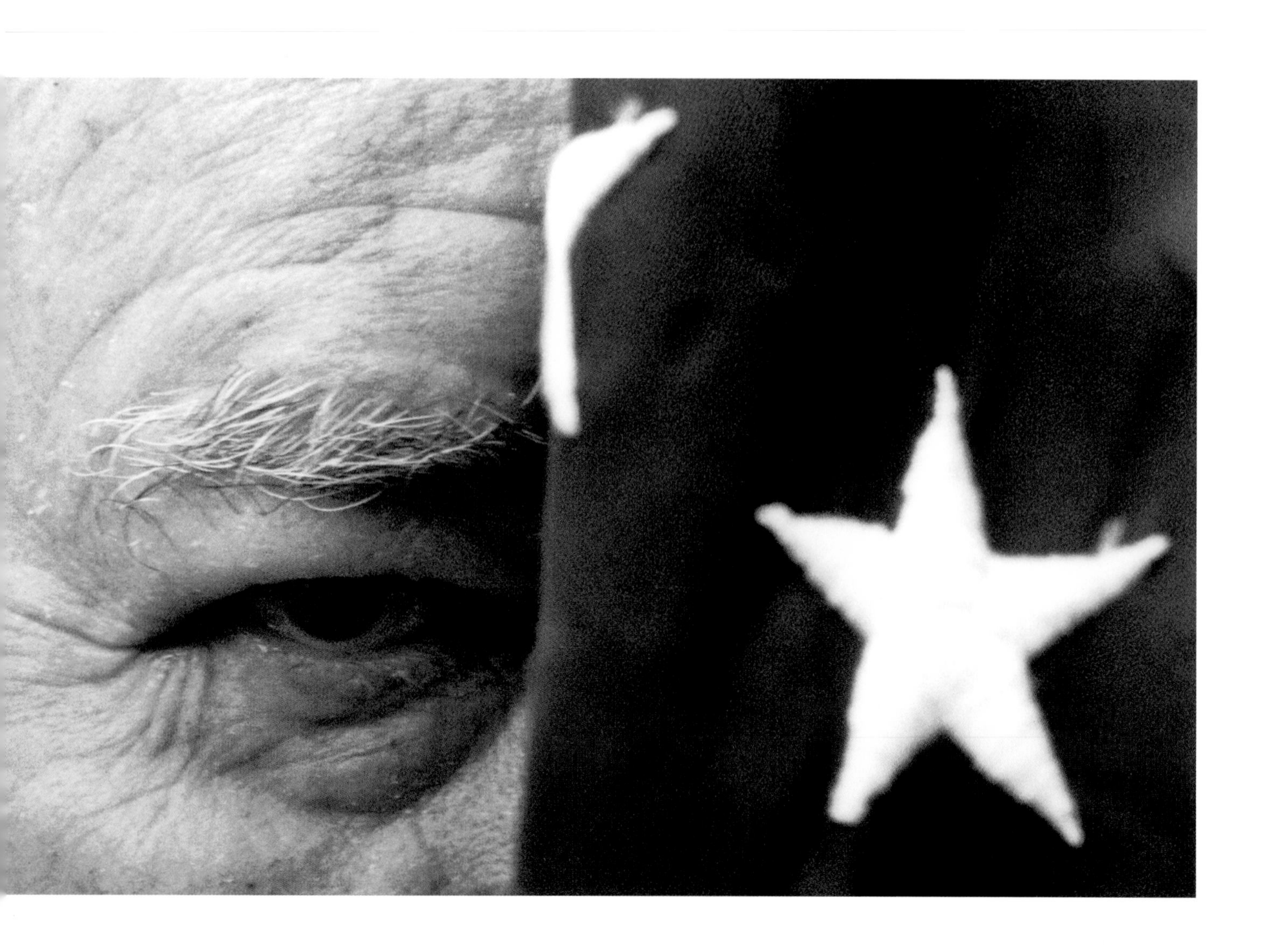

Do you see me?

Mayflies
Emerge alone,
To alight with delicacy
Together.

06/03/99

Couple at Sunset, Carmel Beach, Carmel-by-the-Sea, California 2001

The wind settles.
Snow surrounds the grass.
White clouds
Merge at the margin
Of dead branches fingering the sky.

Trapped water
Hardens in the ditch
Along the track.
Below the cold steel rails
Soft ties pretend to bend
As down trains
Push them periodically apart.

There is no way
To call
Across the intervening years
To where,
At a certain time,
A moment
Beside a warm kitchen,
A family was born,
Or why.

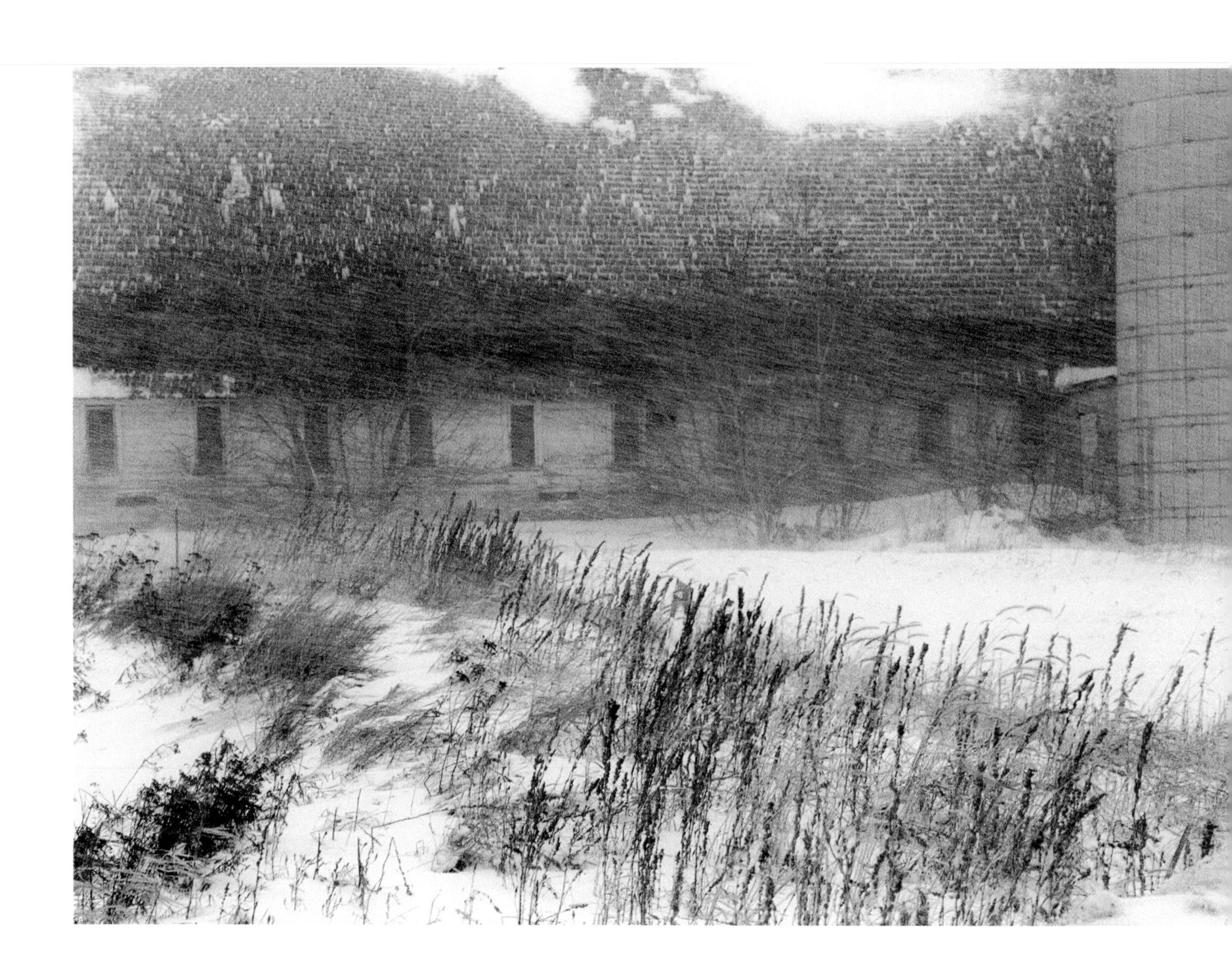

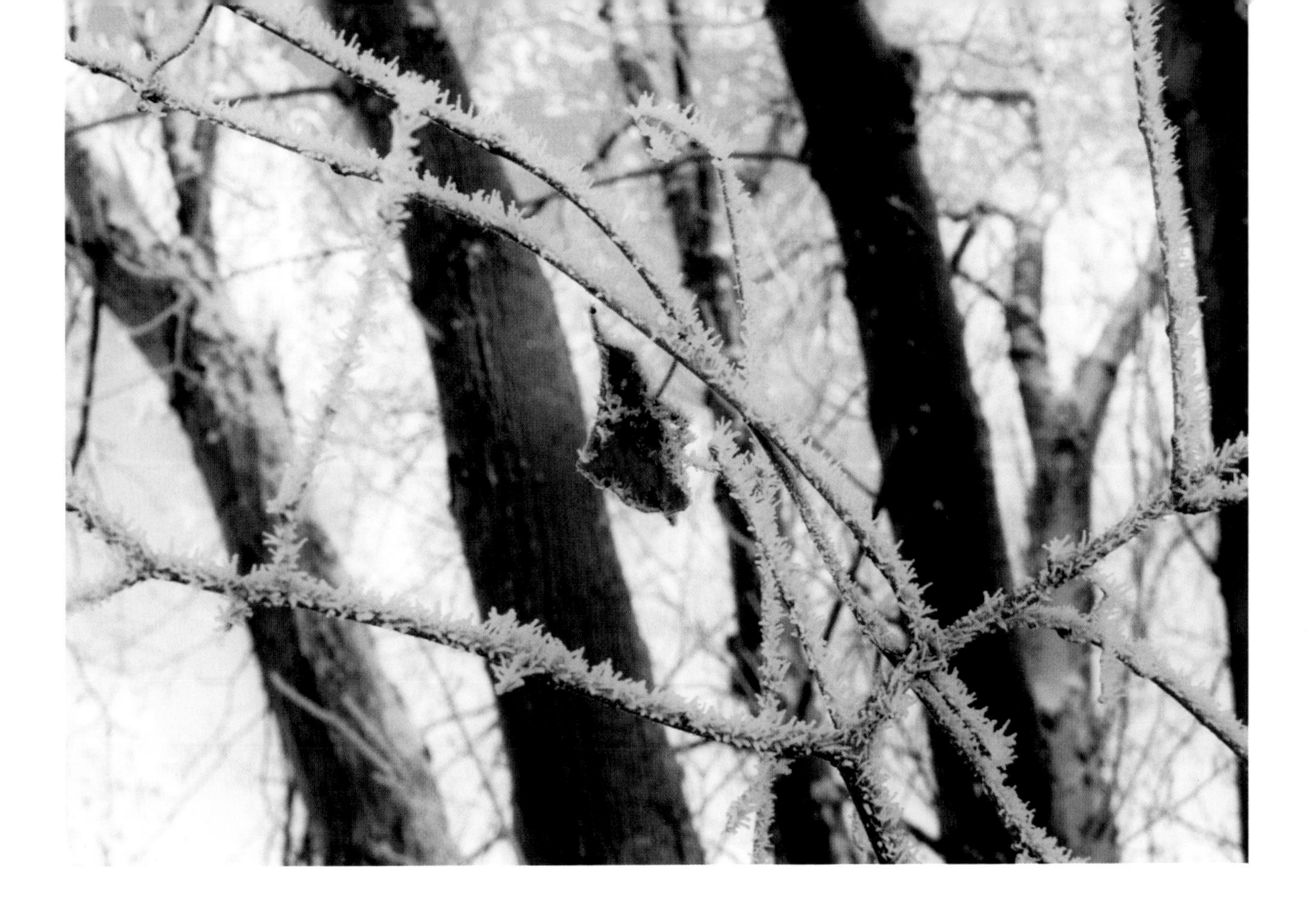

Leaves are falling
Erratically,
Haphazardly,
Tumbling,
Twisting,
Corkscrewing their way to the ground.

Every once in a while,
One leaf slides away,
Gracefully,
Moving down
And across
A cushion of air,
To where it lands,
Sedately.

Leaf, French Rapids, Crow Wing County, Minnesota 1998 | 10/15/01

Good Vibrations
Create new reality
Out of the fertile void.

The wet road
Winds through the dripping trees
Beside telephone lines.

Which goes faster,
My feet upon the slippery clay,
Or words that speed along the wires,
Where no tired eyes
Or grimaces,
Refine the messages?

I can find ways to hide
What I truly think and feel
When I race along
Electronic corridors.

But sitting here,
With you,
At the end of your road,
My life,
You see me in this moment,
Registering the photons
Bouncing from my smiles
And tears.

I had hoped for a reprieve,
A chance to start again
At childhood's end.

We say, "Goodbye,"
And hug each other
One last time.

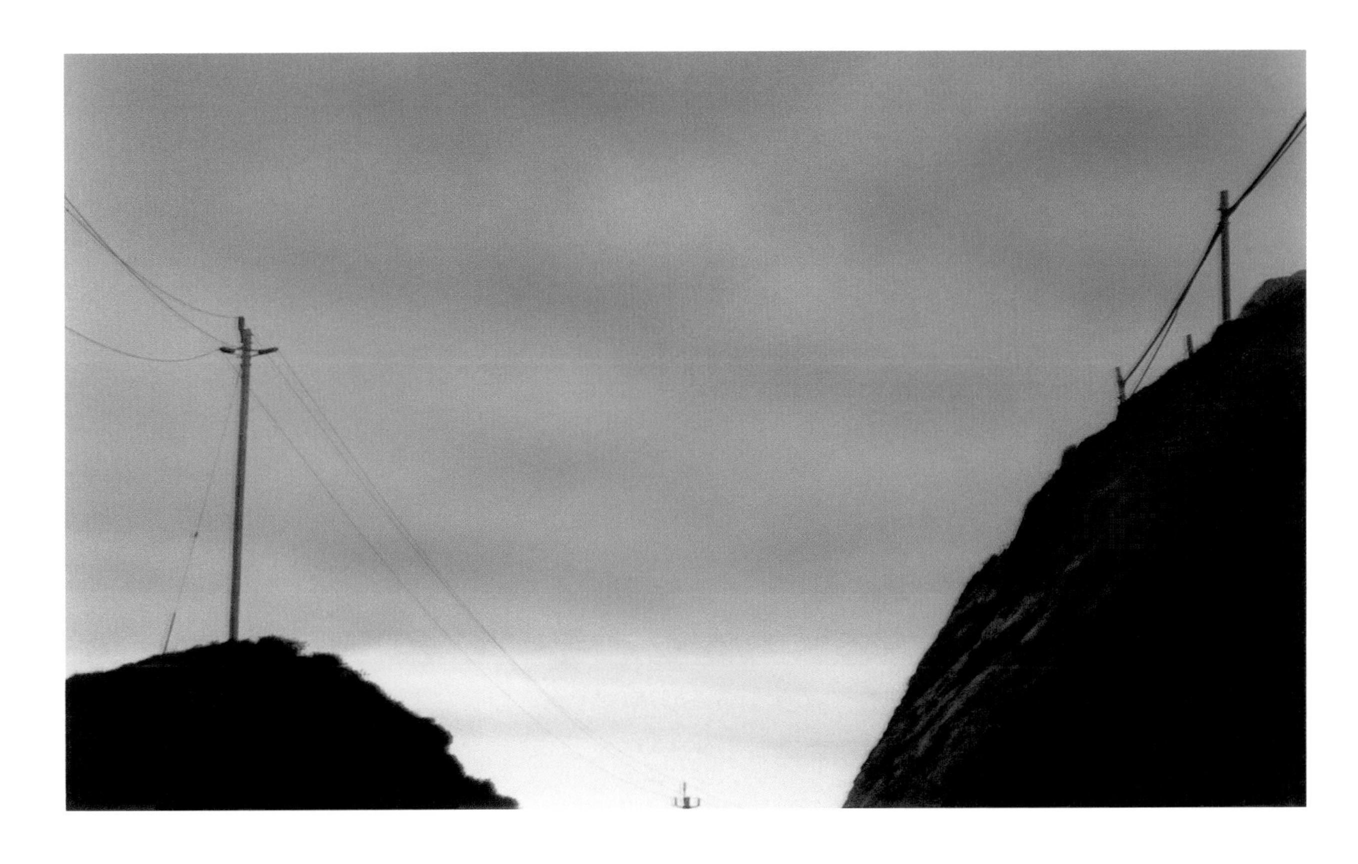

We know what lies ahead,
And remember what once was.

Your love and generosity
Are now a part of me;
Those parts of you
That make me more complete.

Thank you for being,
My friend!

11/07/01

Telephone Lines, Highway 1, South of Carmel-by-the-Sea, California 2001

Our aloe sits alone,
Rimmed with spines,
Protecting its healing powers,
Artfully.

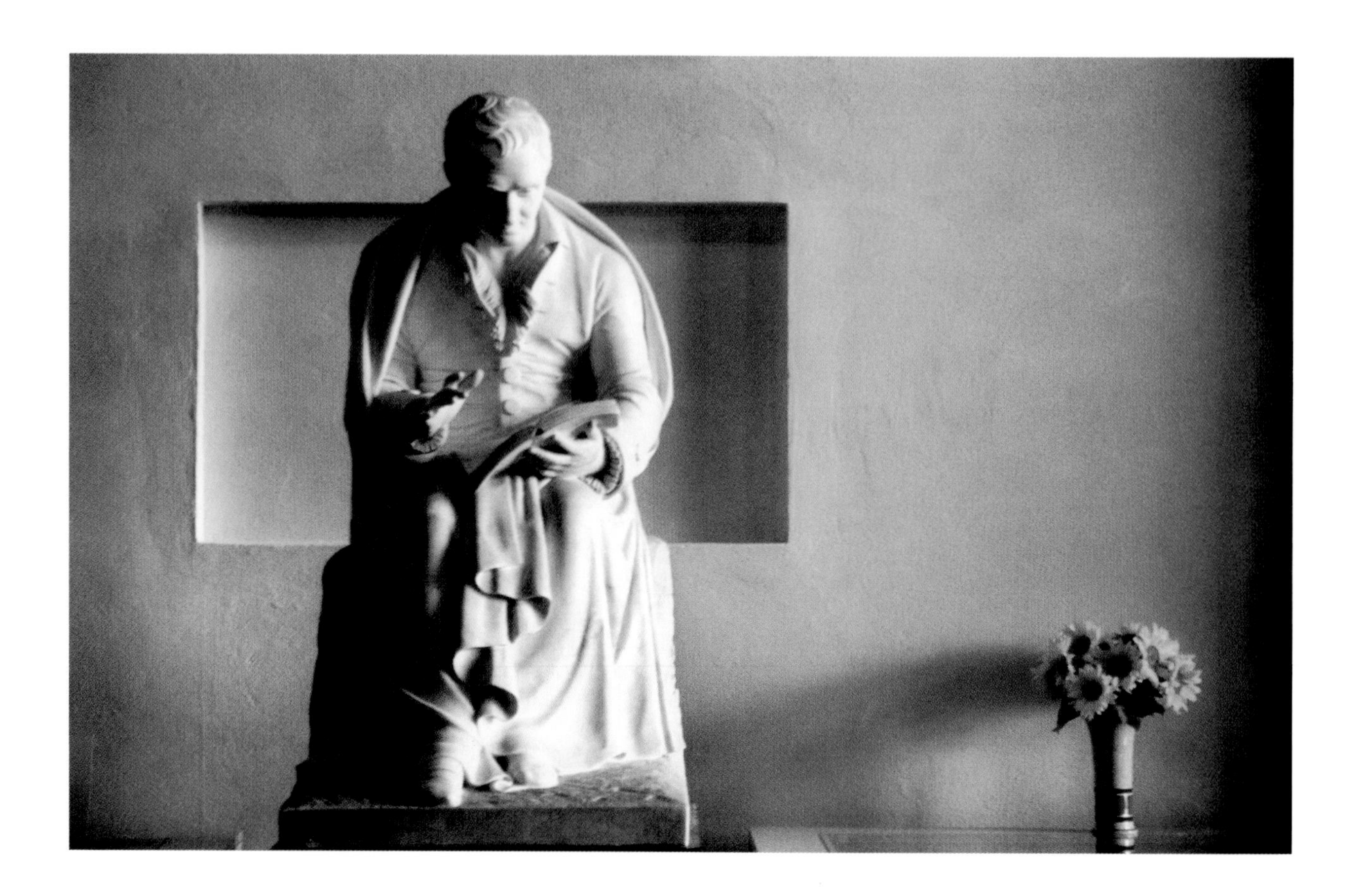

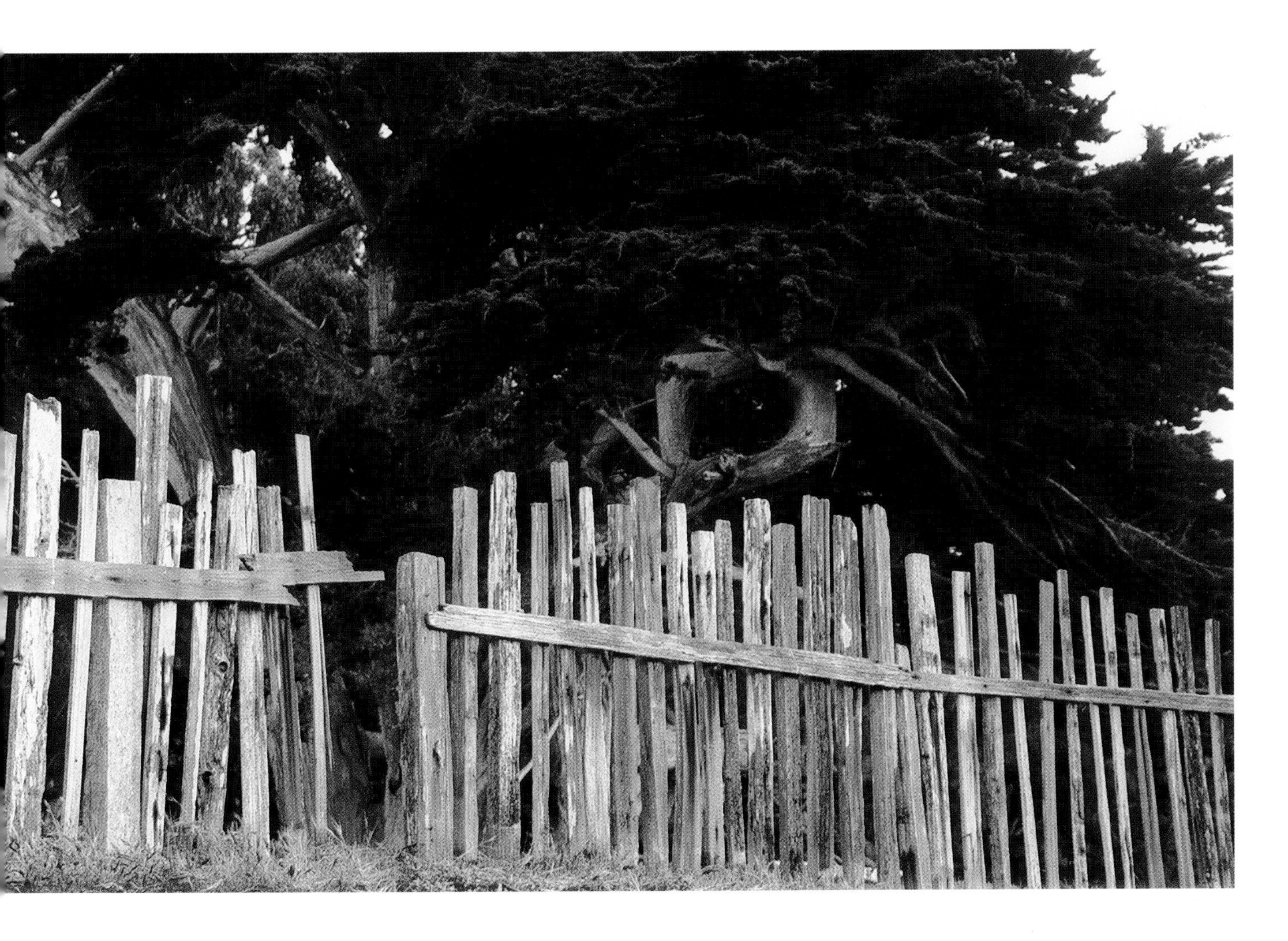

Your world is too small!
How did it get that way?

Your world is the outline
of boundaries you set
When you decided
How to be
Your you.

What was missing
In the microcosm of your life?
What trace element,
Essential for vital living,
Did you lack?

When did you decide
To back away
From the unknown edge,
And settle for safety?

Who told you that the world
was too dangerous,
Too filled with obstacles
That you could never overcome?

Behind your pressured speech,
Your insensitive interruptions,
An energetic intellect is still struggling
To be heard,
Fearful of being forgotten,
Afraid of being,
Overlooked,
Again.

Seaward Fence, Opening, Carmel Bay, California 2001 | 11/15/01

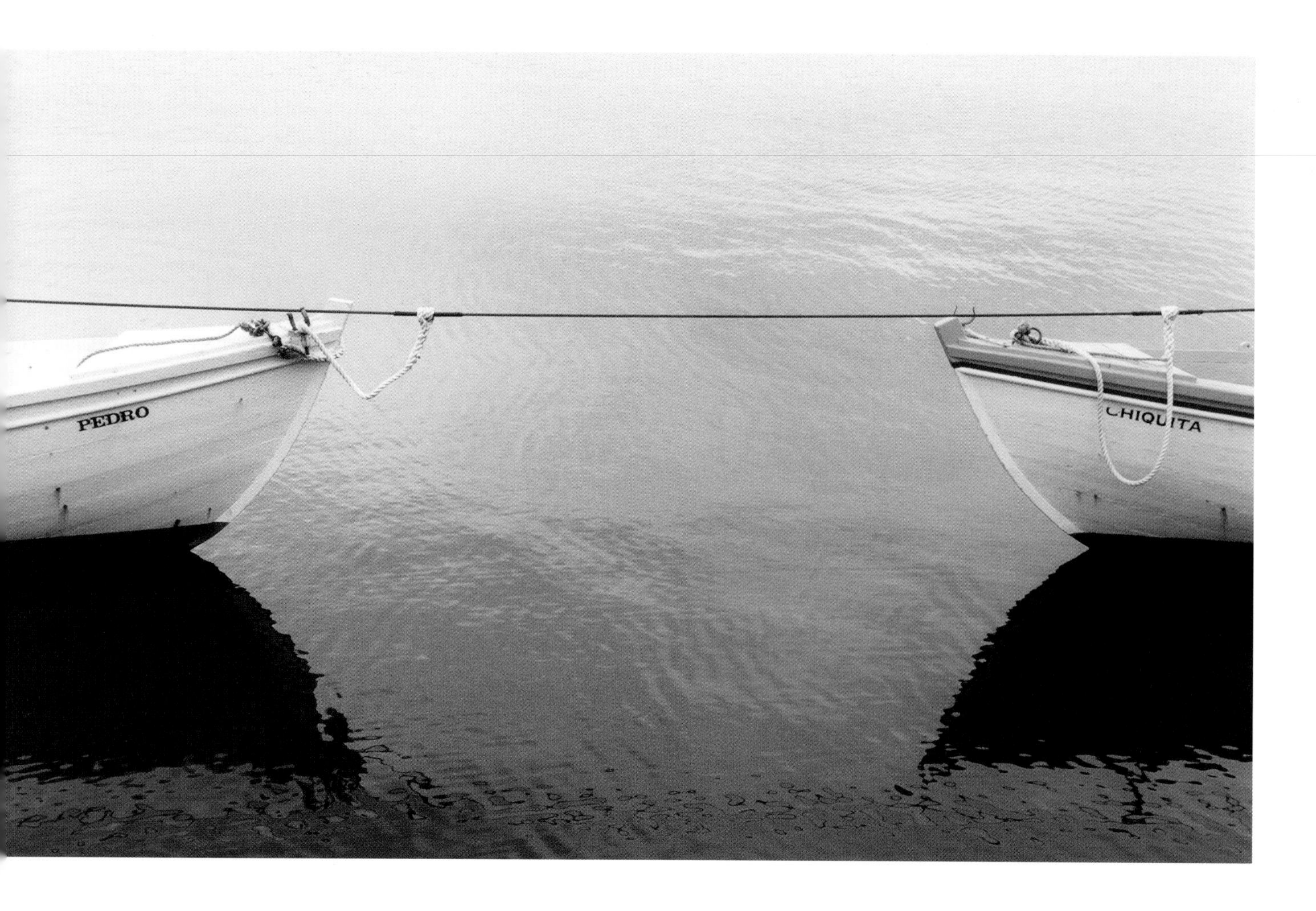

Like the tides,
There are rhythms
Of ebb
And flow
Between us,
From energy
Emerging
Beyond awareness.

Always in touch,
We are closer,
Further apart,
Always in the same ocean
Of mutual awareness,
Moved by energy
Emerging
Beyond awareness,
Again
And
Again.

Unresolved, Mystic River, Mystic, Connecticut 1998 | 06/22/98

Unapparent weakness
In the heart of the tree
Made it break,
Instead of bending,
Unexpectedly.

In the midst
Of other silent trees,
It broke,
Pouring out its hurt
Where no one heard
And no one spoke.

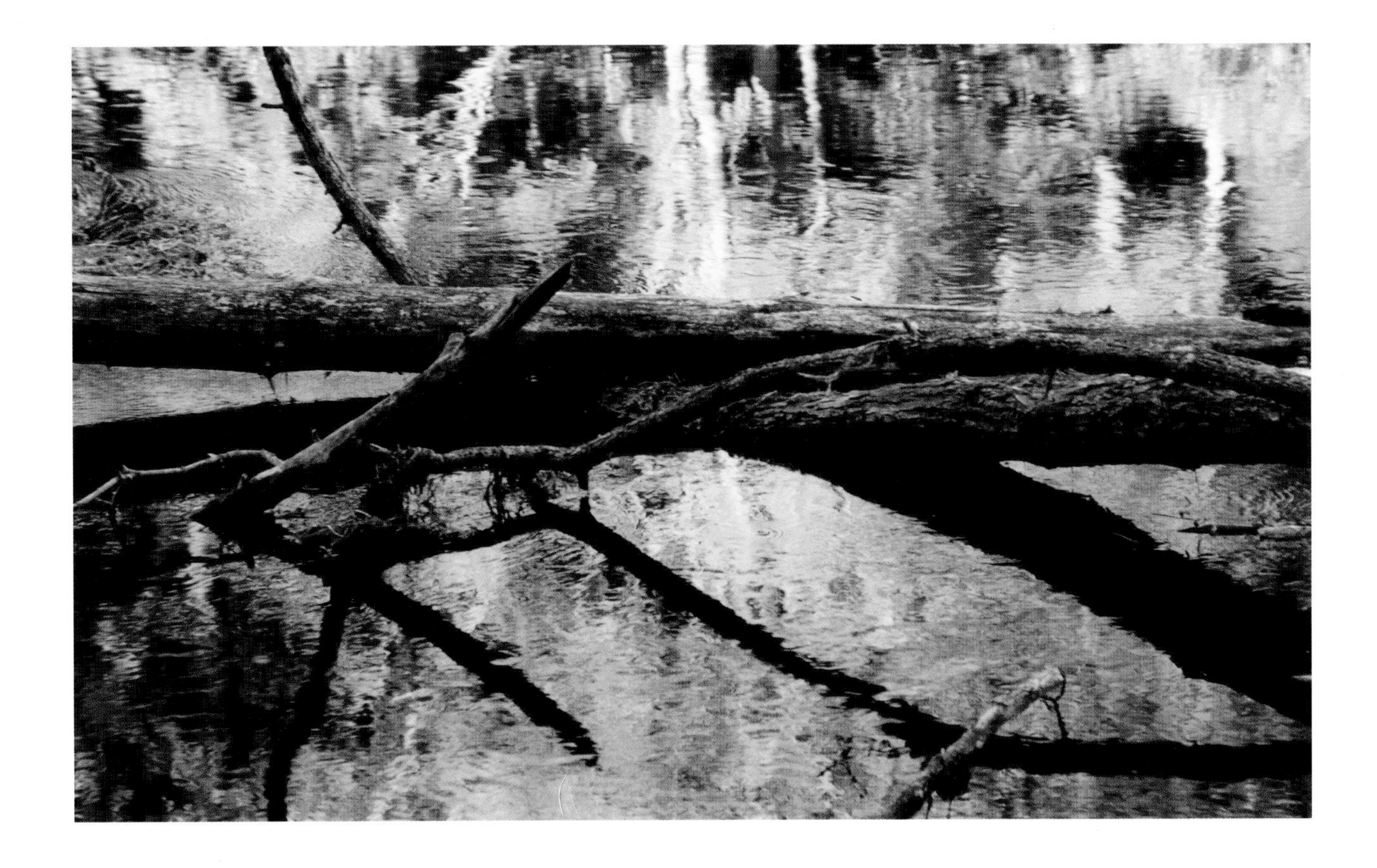

We stand at the mirror, for a moment,
Our images together, flat, untouchable, unreachable;
Like high music straining to break up,
Around the boundaries of sound,
Edged by oval emptiness
And silence slit by strings.
The mirror is a merger,
The reflection of a hope,
Reality caught for a moment
In the flat mass of the glass.

I used to be afraid in barbershops
Of getting caught and ultimately lost
In fading images,
Diminishing in two directions.

I have a new respect for mirrors now,
And my roughskin chin
And I know I will not be lost,
Forever.

Blue shadows merge in snowlight white.
Footprints plot their paths,
And shadows leave their mark.
Snow and salt and cars of cavernous emptiness
Stretch pebbled shadows along uneven crusts of blown snow.
Purple shadows of trees are scattered and shattered on petite, plowflung peaks.
They stand aside for an instant
Where grey shadows of people override
And distance disappears.

Words are born in warm wombs,
Through lips that pull and push apart,
By tongues that touch as they explore the way words soften space between lovers,
—and there is more, and always more.

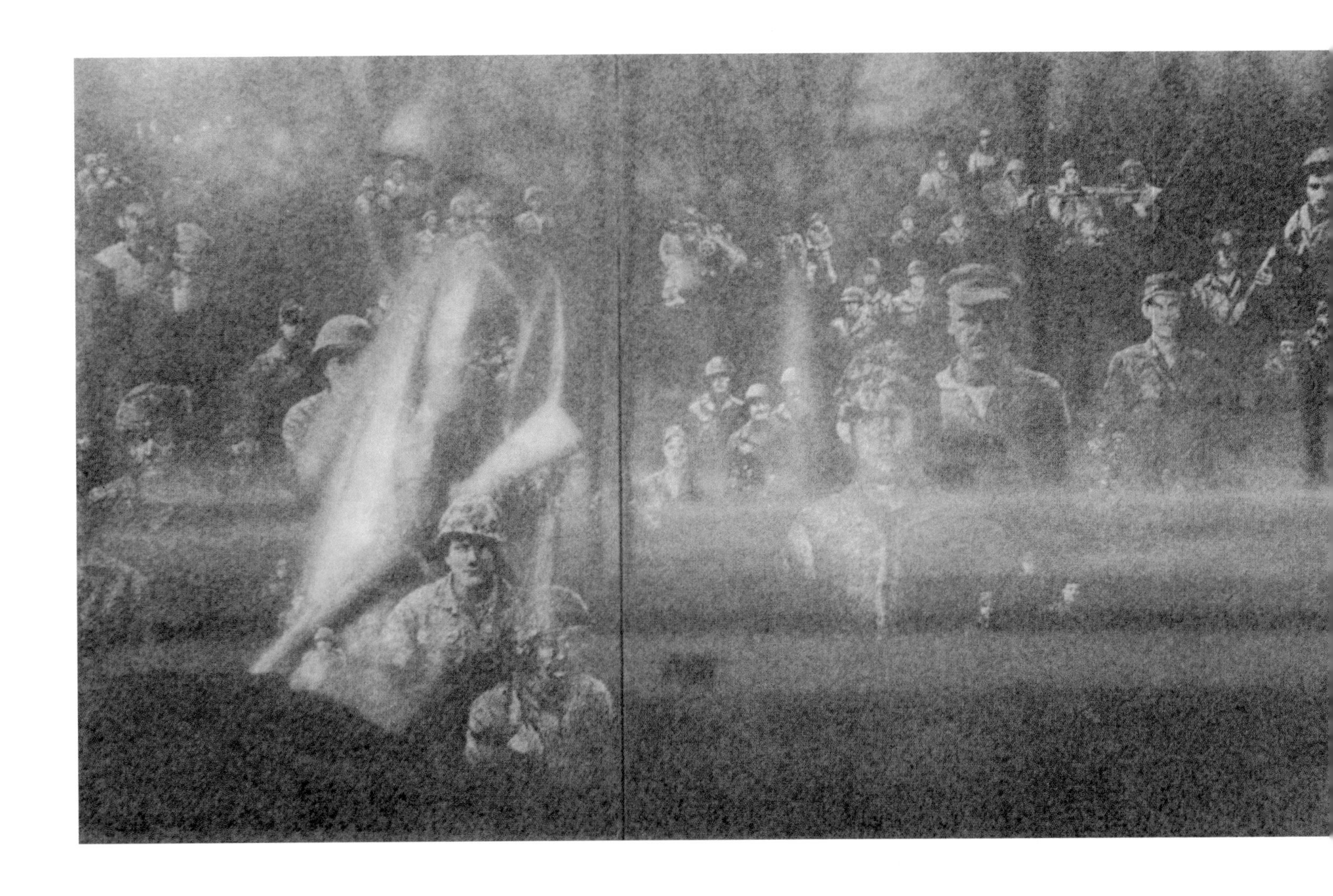

01/28/70 | *At the Mirror,* Korean War Memorial, Washington, D.C. 2000

per luce tuam videmus

So much depends on seeing,
That even the blind
Are sometimes accused
Of "second sight."

From time to time,
An insensate fog
Or mist,
Emerges in my mind.

Then,
What I want to see
Is caught in particulate light,
Creating subtle contrasts
Of what I am
With what I want to be.

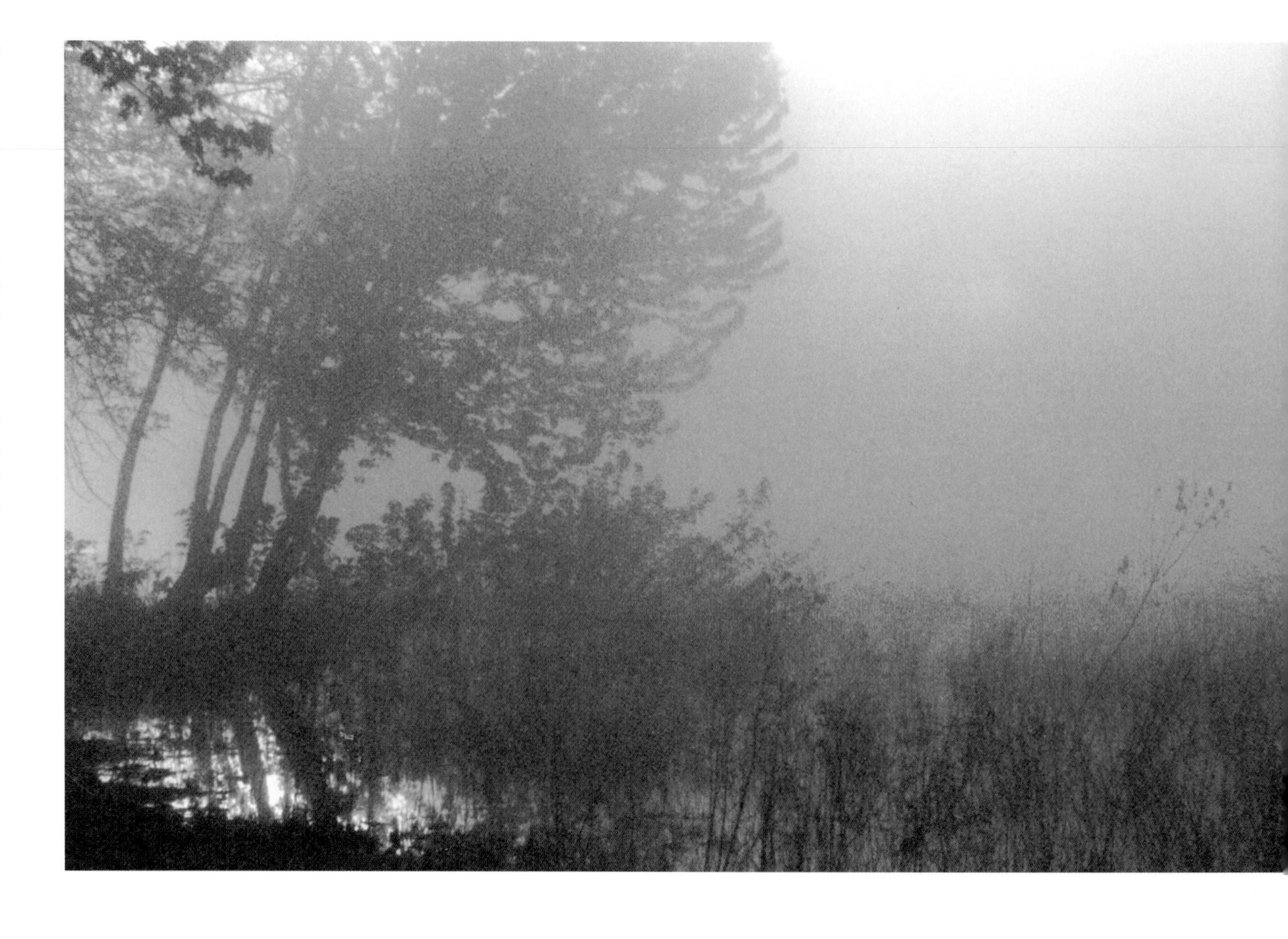

11/13/01

East Light, Boom Lake, Brainerd, Minnesota 1994

The wind,
Rushing through the trees,
Scraping up the snow
As it skims across the lake,
May wipe my words away
As soon as I begin to speak.

So listen
Carefully,
And I,
In my time,
will finally
Let you hear your voice
Reverberate
In mine.

We have fallen into Fall.
The dark
Is coming
Earlier
This year.

It was there,
This morning,
A piece of poem,
Just three lines,
Fully formed,
Ready to be written.

But they escaped.
Lost.
Gone.

Perhaps they lie
Like my ancestors
In unmarked graves,
Waiting for a resurrection
That might,
Or might not
Come.

Perhaps they will emerge
Without warning
In a dream,
A paragraph,
An essay,
Or the story of a soul
Wrapped in mystery,
Trapped in myth,
Waiting for a voice
To find them,
Again.

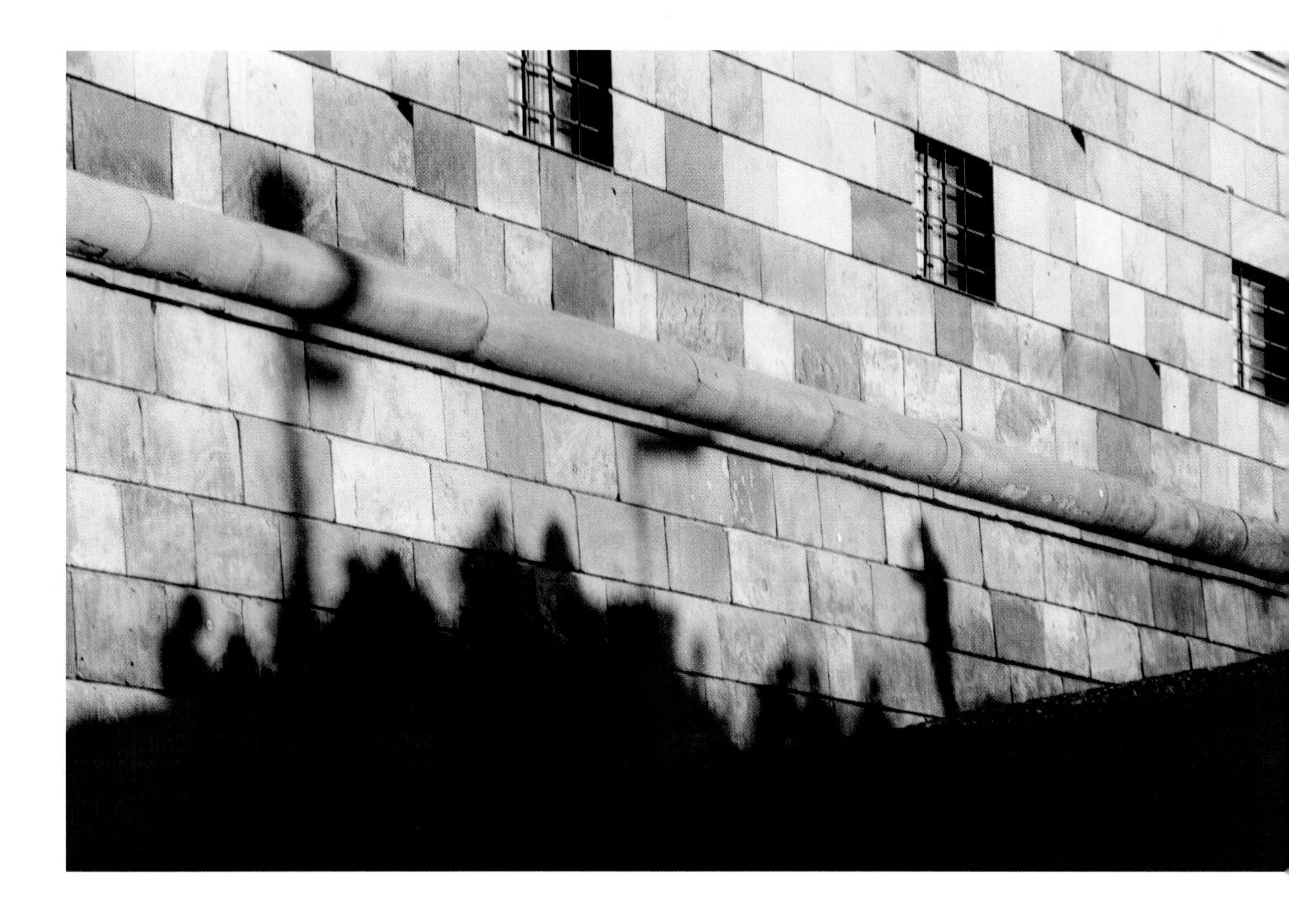

03/04/99

Waiting Shadows, King's Palace, Stockholm, Sweden 1997

Trees, Spring, Bay Lake Township, Minnesota 1995

Inverted ice dream cones
Of energy,
Groping through gravel
To security,
They stand tall
Along the edge
Of my responsibility.

Late day sun
Warms one side,
Creating great black shadows
Against a growing green.

Supported by the snow
And brown dead drying leaves,
They wait,
They wish for nothing
More
Than Spring
To come,
Again.

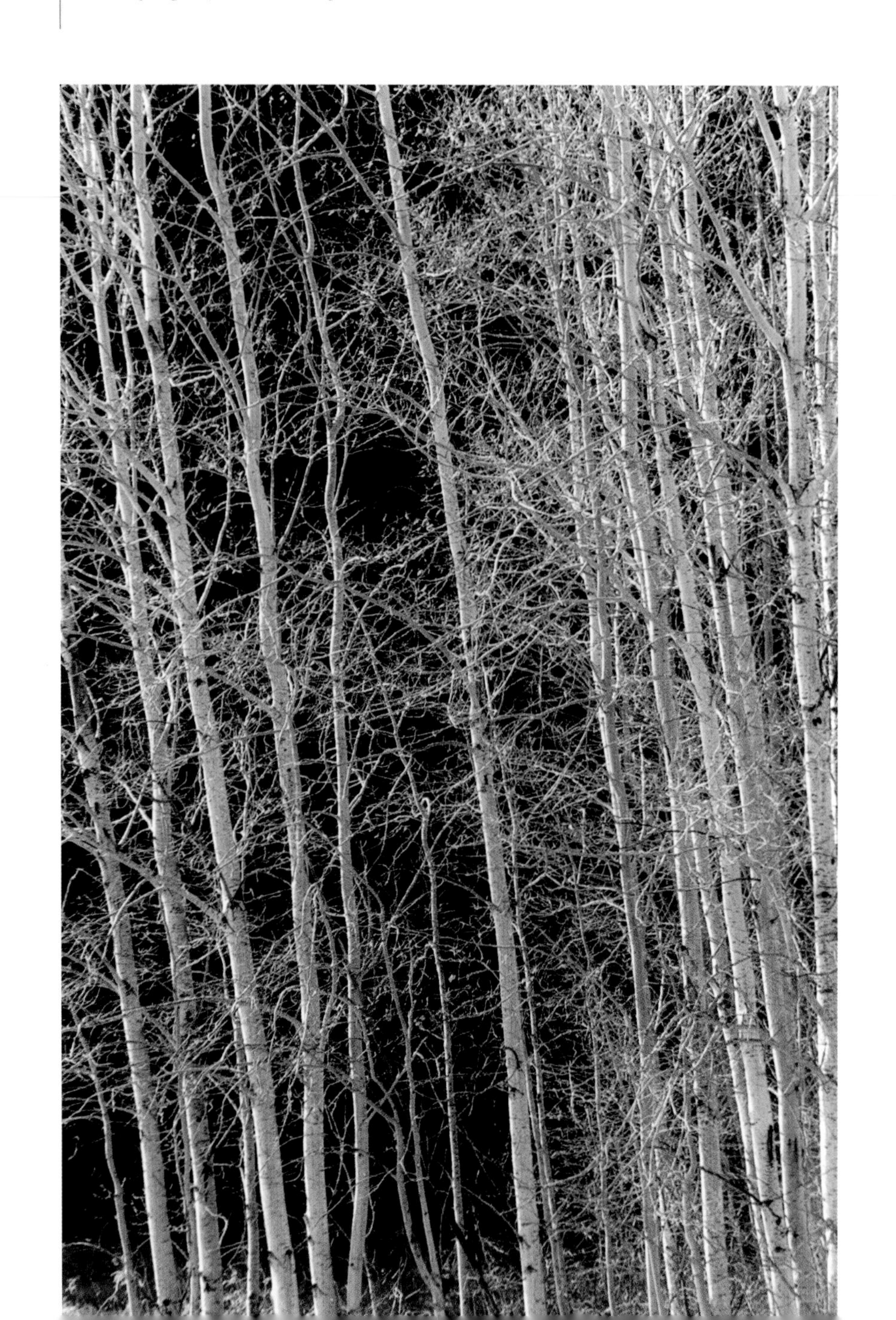

I'm hiding in the underbrush of words . . .
There's no place else to go . . .
I'm afraid to go again . . .
I will still be running when I die . . .

Passage, Georgetown, Washington, D.C. 2000 | 07/21/70

Shrouded Sun, Gull River Basin, Crow Wing County, Minnesota 1996

The air is thin,
And empty now.
The last departing flight
Is long since
Out of sight,
And only empty
Shreds of clouds
Close in upon
The coming night.

The shrouded sun
Emerges weakly
Underneath its fading shadows,
Striking off
A fragmented spectrum,
But not enough
To make
A rainbow
Or a bend.

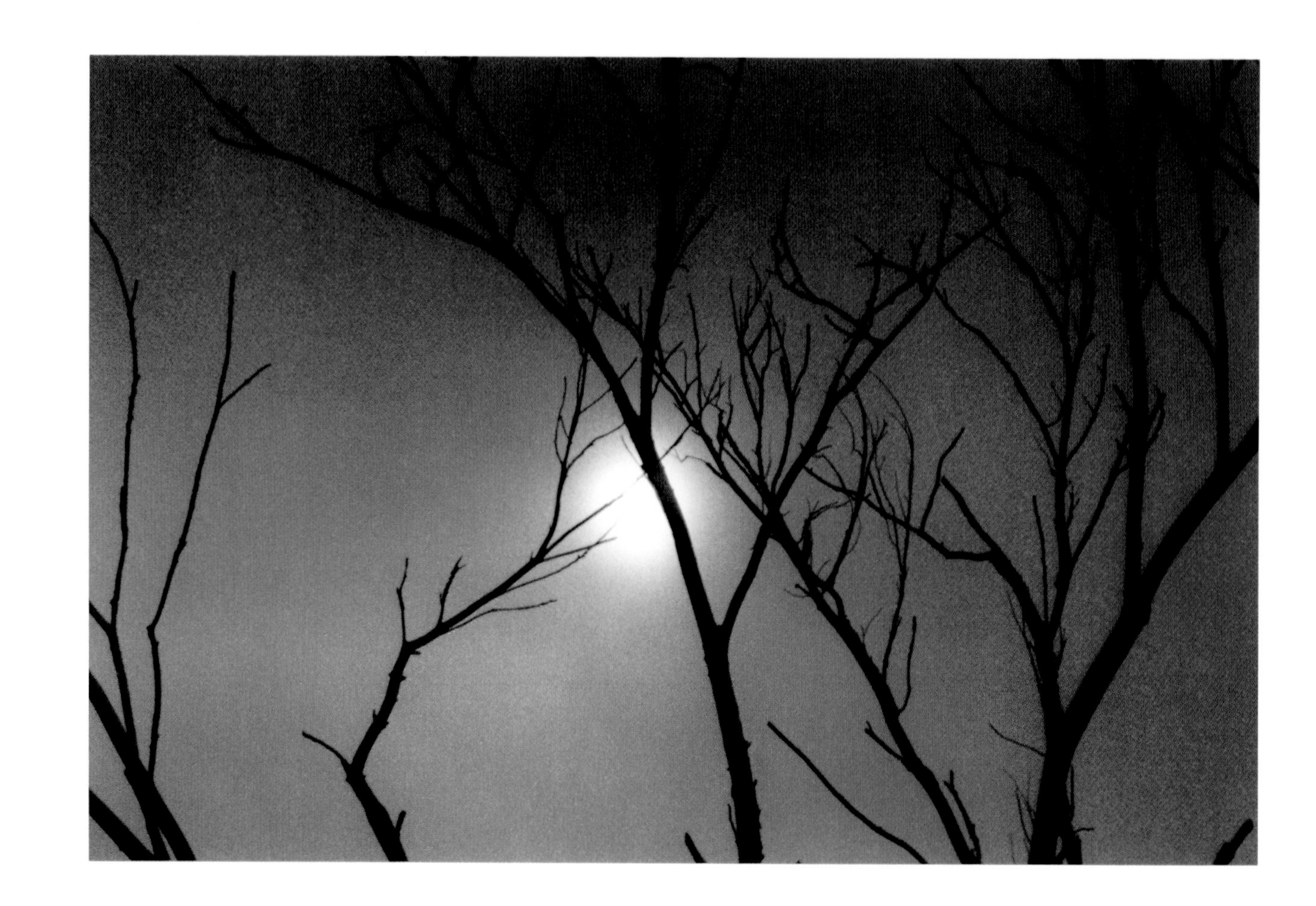

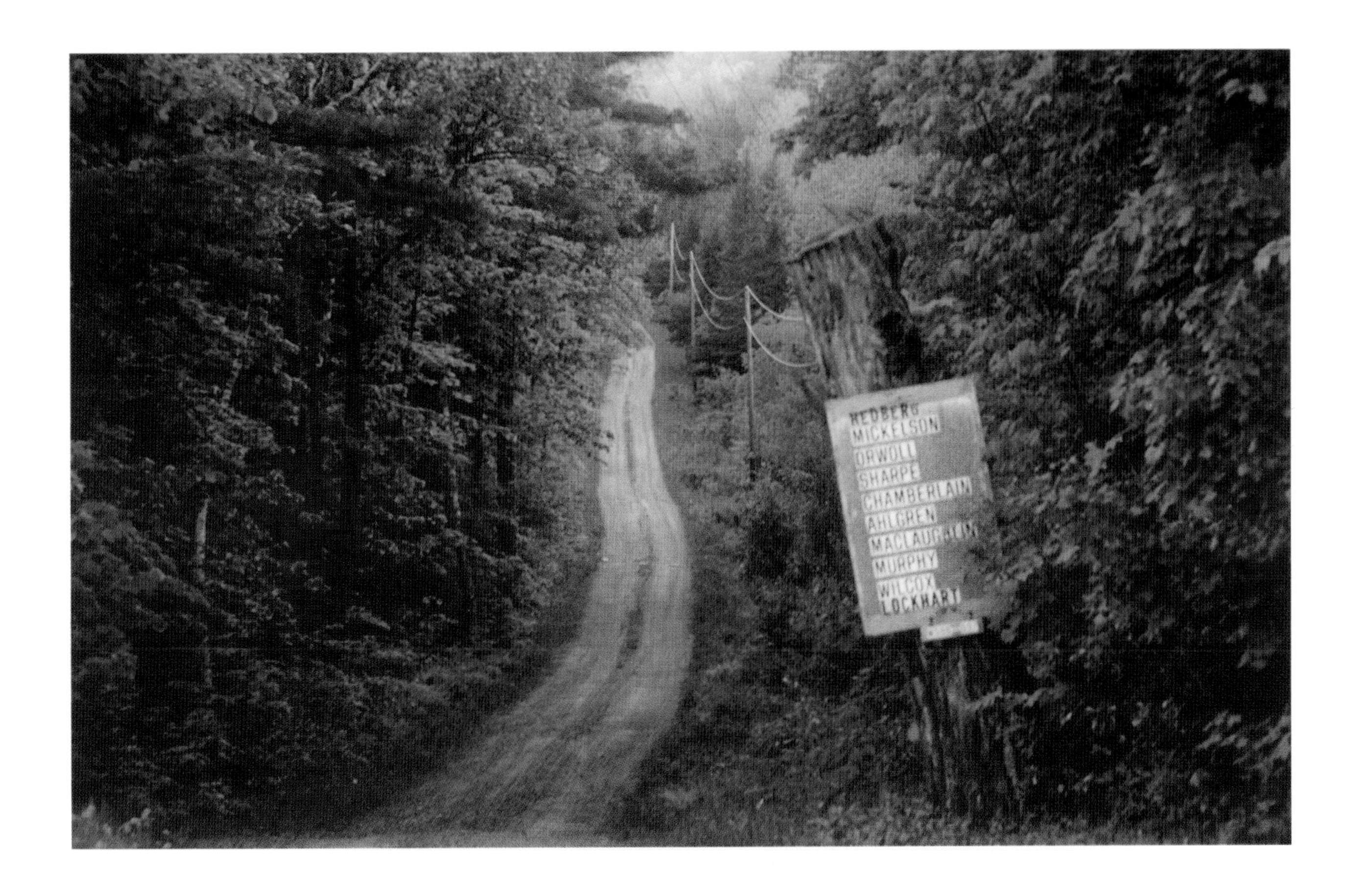

I am a part
Of what is now
Evolving here:
The grey, warm rain
    Dripping,
    After being caught by trees,
    Stopped
    In flat sheets,
    In shallow pans of clay
    Along barely rutted paths
    Between softening bricks
    And flaking,
    Whitened,
    Rotting
    Wood.

The rain that wets beneath dried grass
The blind burrowing of worms,
Clouds the eyes of birds and squirrels
    Searching for a soft,
    Warm
    Place
    To be.

Dampened Road, Bay Lake Township, Minnesota 1993 | 02/15/90

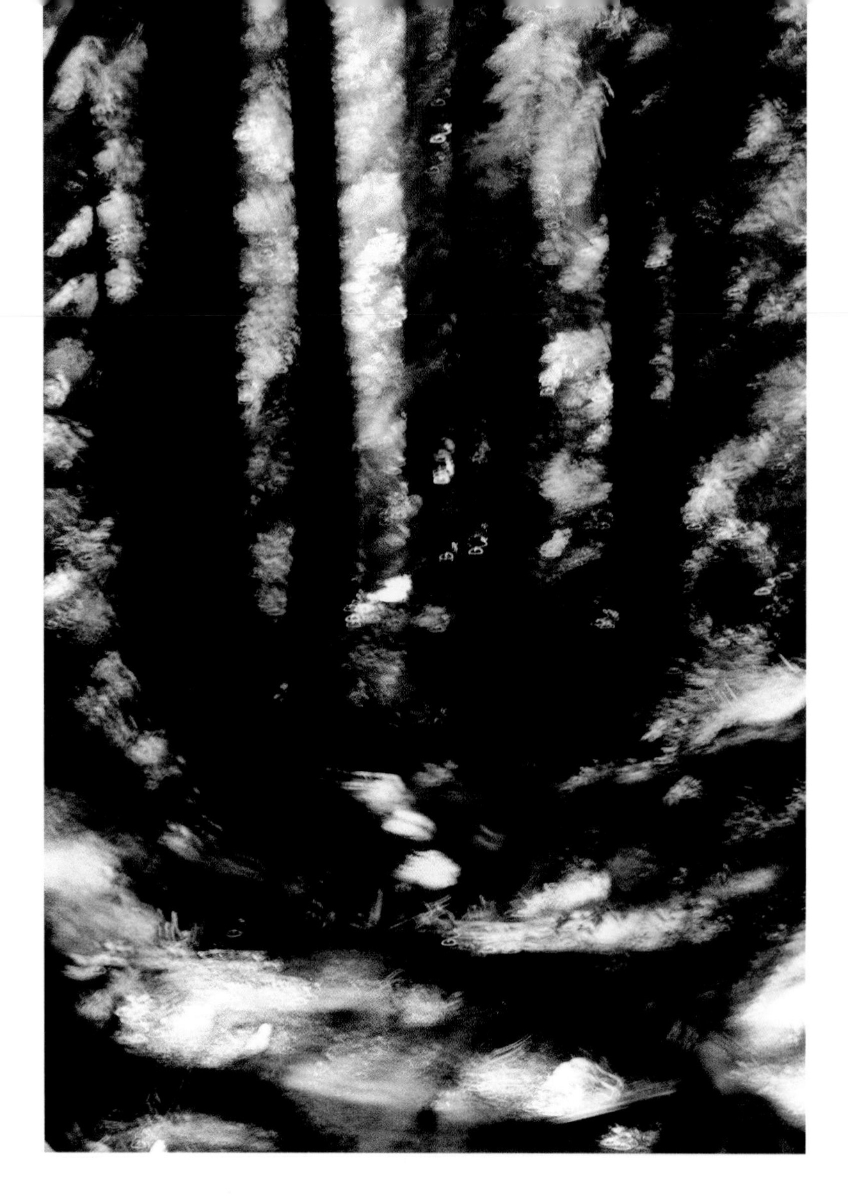

I wish to walk the ferny glens of time,
Between the narrowed pinions
of sharp shaley heights;
To find around each craggy bend
a shaft of sunlight
Straightened and cradled
through patterns of leaves
After its desolate journey
Through the bitterness of space.

Infinity, Big Sur, California 2001 | 11/26/63

Time
Is the river
In which
All is.

Leaves fall,
Trees die,
To keep the forest
Alive.

Was the leaf
I saw
Fall
Aware of its own
Gravity?

Memories are reflections
Of fragments
Caught in an instant,
Forever.

Eternal life
Is stringing threads
Of DNA
Across time.

We may be different,
But we are
So much
Alike!

What flows beneath,
Or moves above,
Is there,
Instantly!

"Each person is meant to represent humanity, in his own way!"

—Friedrich Daniel Ernst Schleiermacher

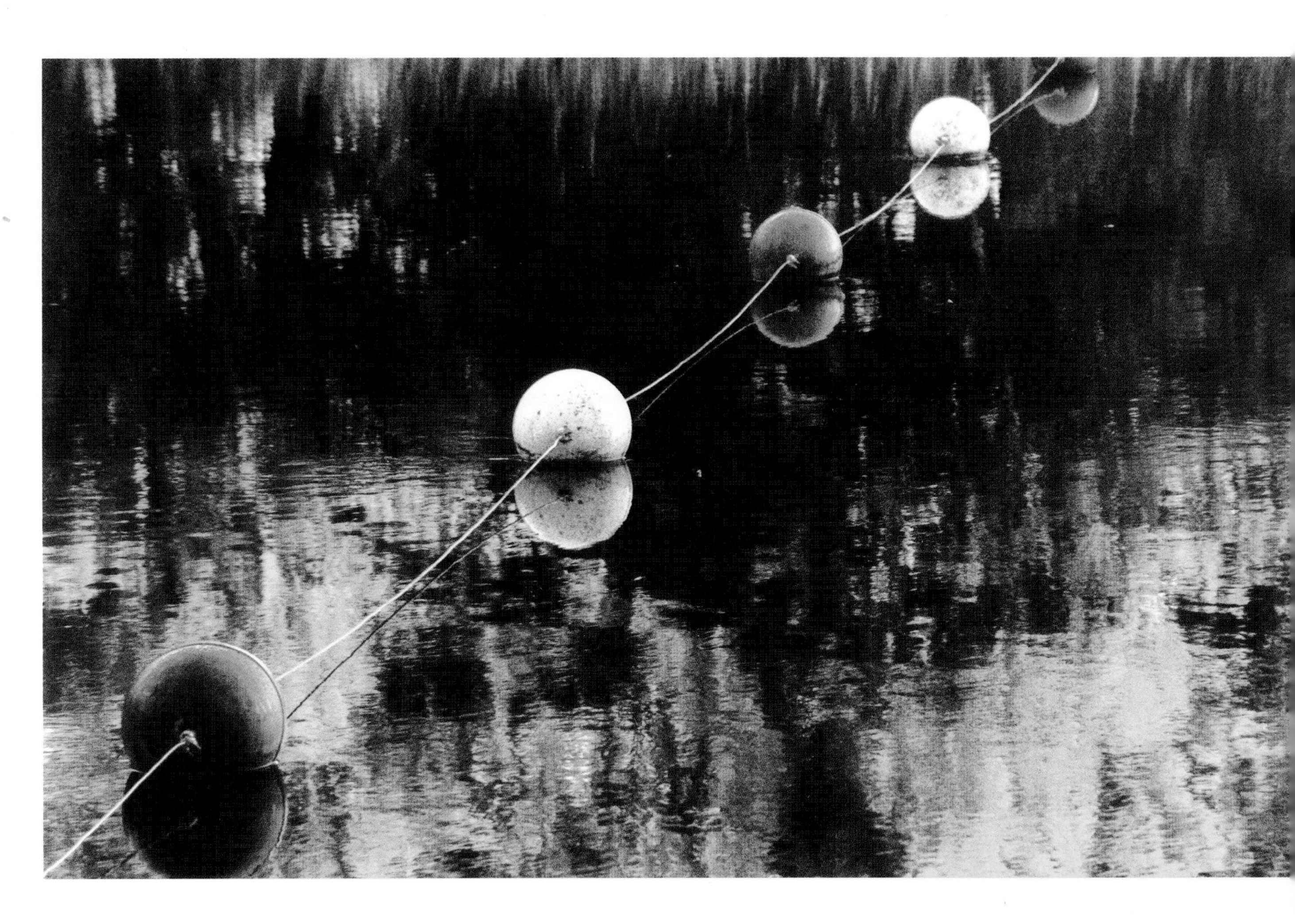

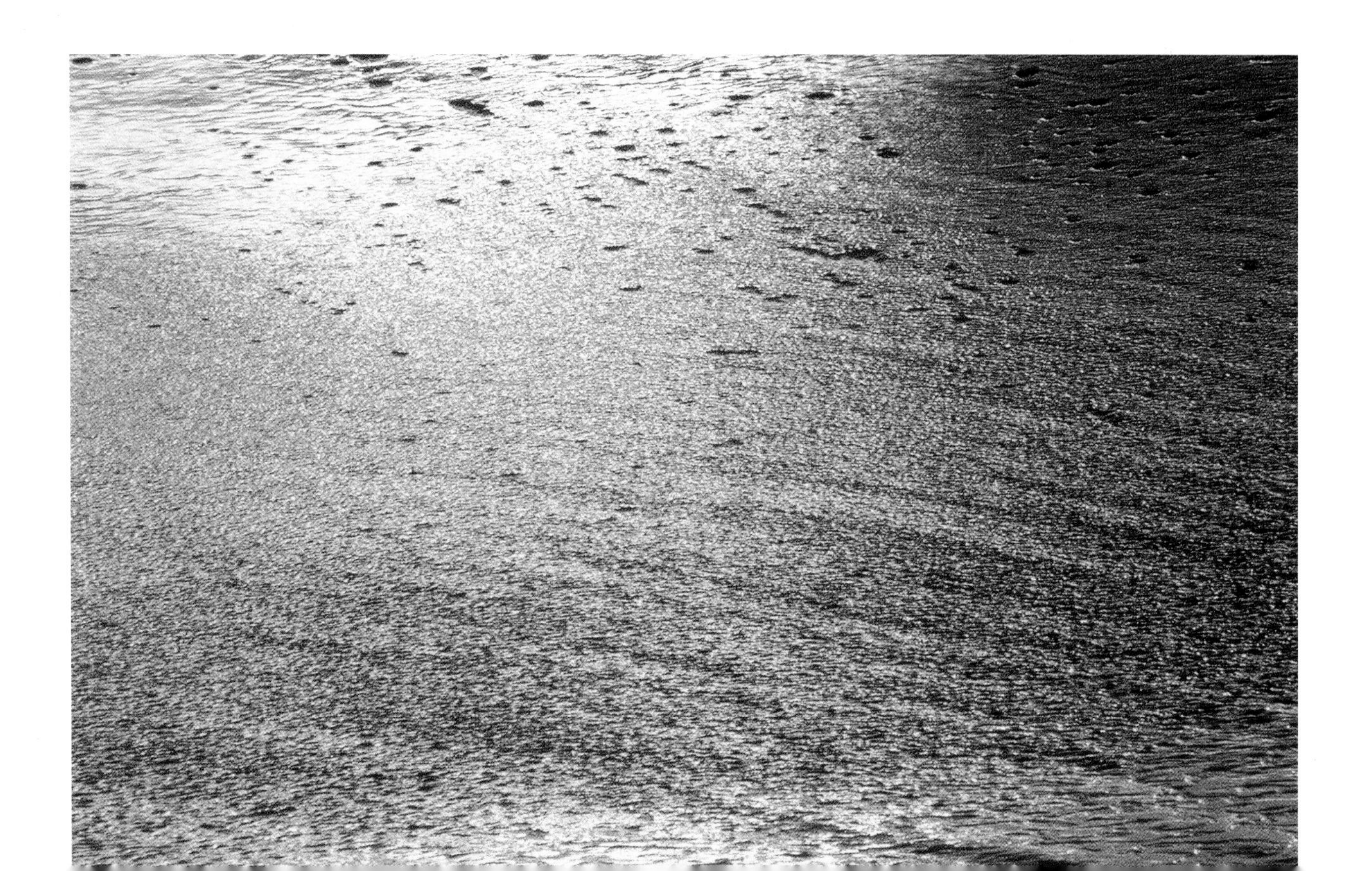

All seconds,
Minutes,
Hours,
Days,
Are equidistant
From infinity.

My boat heels
Before the wind,
Away from its wake,
And into great grey.

06/22/82 | *Boat, Becalmed,* Near Victoria, British Columbia 1995

Rafts of wild ducks,
Born in different places,
Gather here together,
And leave here,
Together.

They stopped for a while,
To husband energy,
I suppose;
To gather what they could
Of rice from a nearby slough
Or tender shoots from submerged plants.

What makes them want to be here,
Together?
Leave together?

What is it in the spiral twists,
The helical turns of their genes,
That makes them want to cluster,
Then head off,
In the same direction?

Is it the same with you and me,
On a more self-conscious scale?

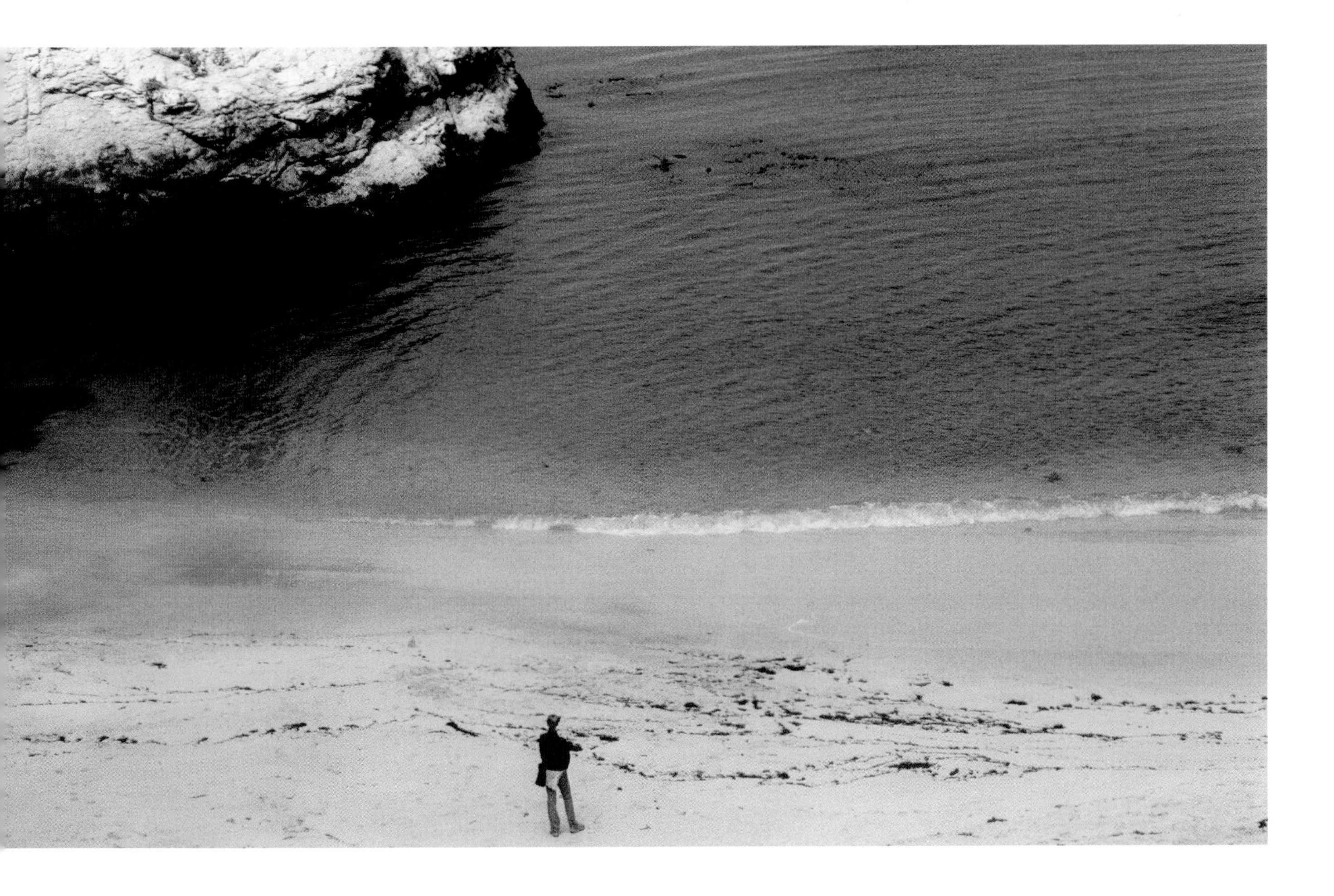

“No man is an island, entire of itself;
Every man is a piece of the continent.”

—*John Donne,* Devotions, 1624

We needn’t plumb the bottom of a bay,
Nor sound the features of the canyons
in the sea,
To know that whatever water hides,
Is of one piece,
Below.

Images and metaphors
Are empty,
Useless,
When I try to realize
How you and I are alike,
Different,
Connected,
Separate,
Together,
Apart.

How can we ever
Become close?

By holding hands?
To eat,
We have to pull away.

By making love?
To dress ourselves
Or go to sleep,
We have to pull away.

Can my words dissolve the distance,
Somehow,
And each of us come to know
Something of the same thing
Of which we are a part,
And always were?

Figure, China Cove, Point Lobos, California 2001 | 10/26/01

Not from a grain of mustard seed
But a thin slice of thistle spawn
You arose.

Some resurrection!

Dying in cold clay,
Surrounded by a stand of trees,
Under overhanging grasses
You found a place to be
And grow!

Now taller than I am,
Your lower leaves are bare,
Barren and brown.

Your puff-pot heads
Strain toward the evening sun,
Away from the woods
Approaching from the rear.

For how long?

Will the coming frost
Destroy the more of you
And snowloads bend your branches
Back to the ground
Where you began?

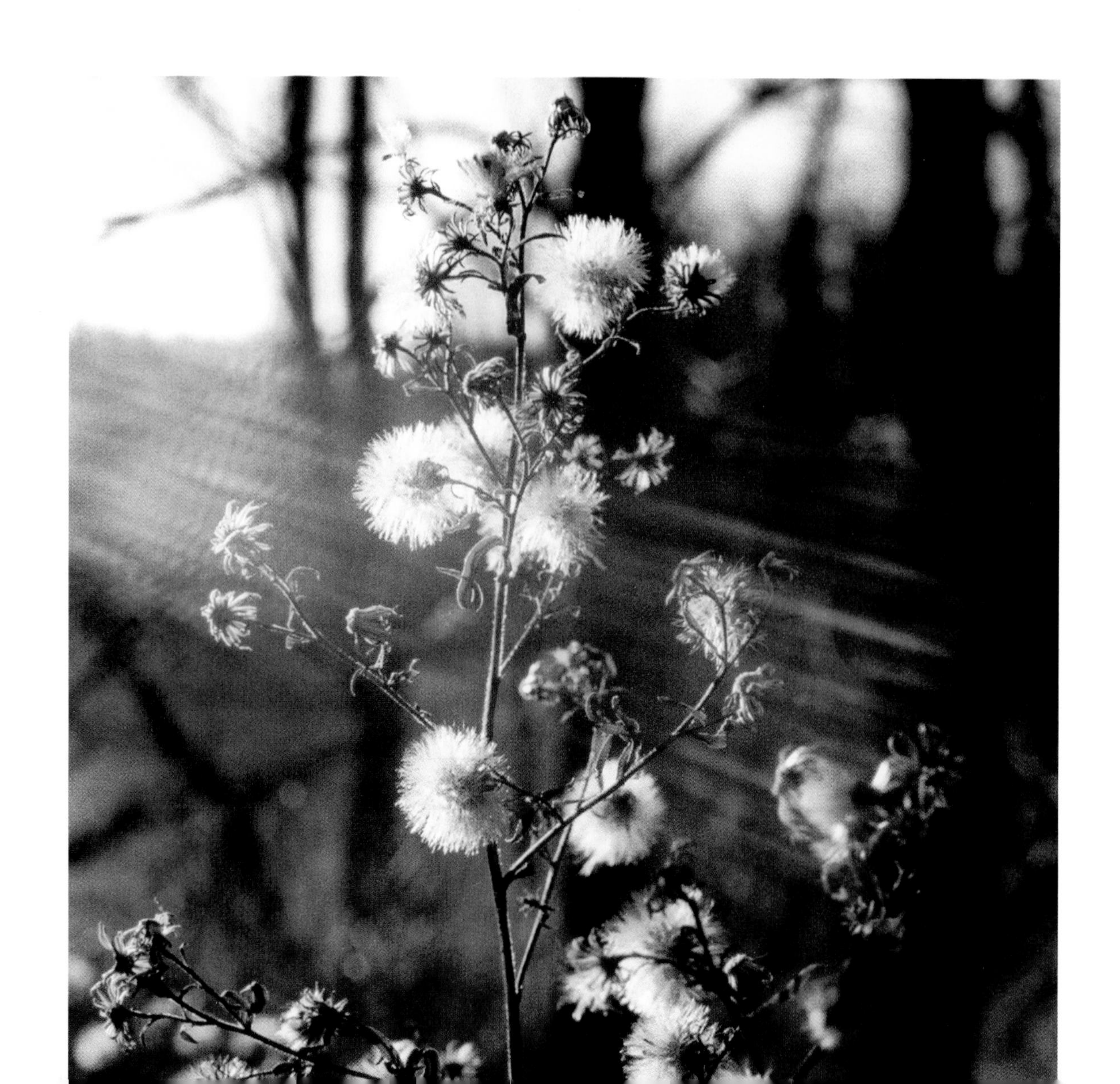

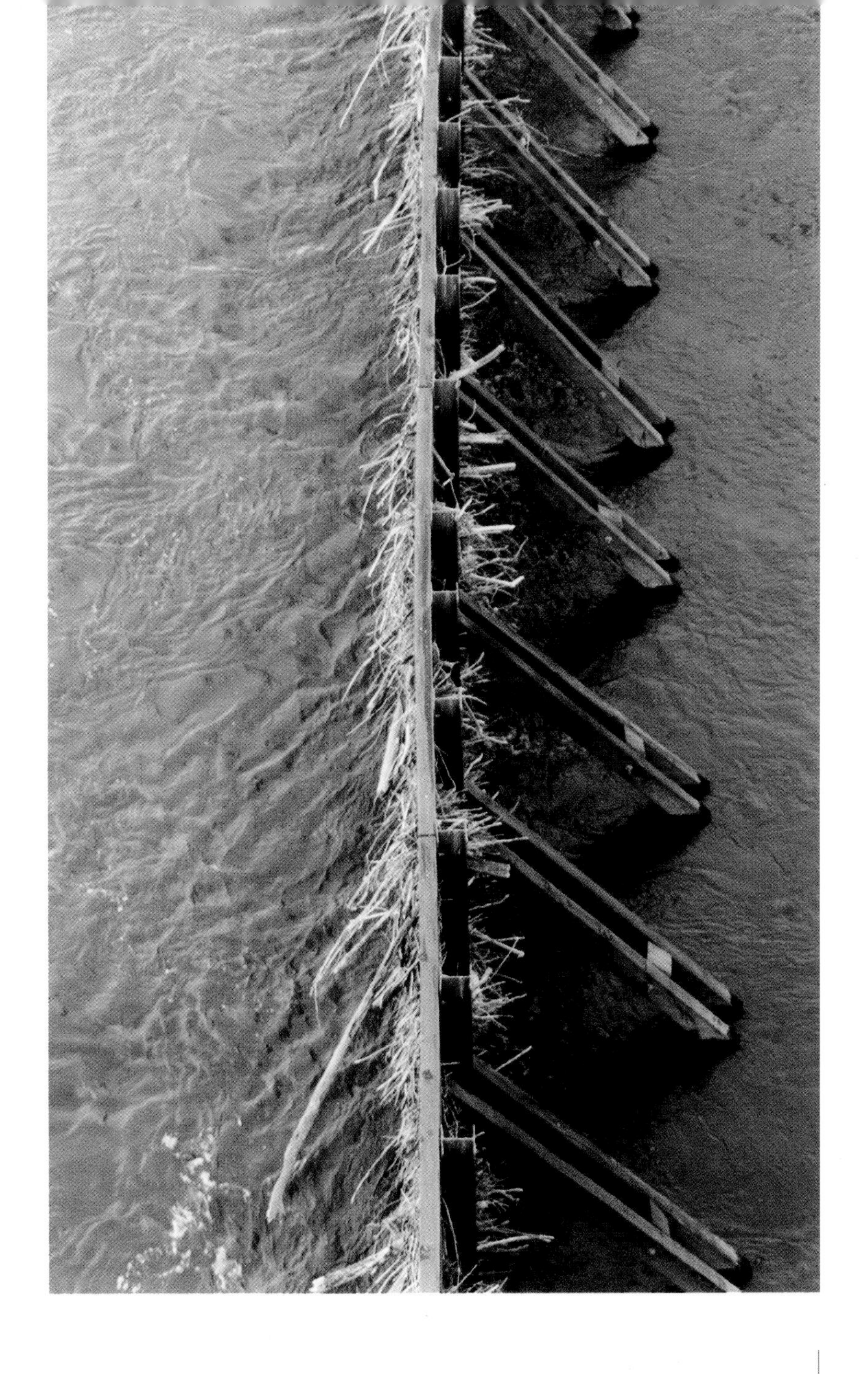

Somebody
Put the pilings there,
Created the cribbing,
But why?

homo faber,
Man the maker always changes things,
Leaving wistful clues,
Cues to think again
About what we do
And why:

Not only do we rearrange the world,
We have the wit and wisdom
To ask the question
"Why?"

Barrier, Mississippi River, St. Paul, Minnesota 2000 | 10/27/01

Evening Tide, Carmel Beach, Carmel-by-the-Sea, California 2001 | 01/04/98

There were those songs
My mother
Never got to sing.

She had a lovely voice,
Soprano,
I suppose,
That stayed on pitch
And strong
Until she was seventy
Or more.

She loved to sing,
And lost herself
Among the ups
And downs
Of notes and rhythms
Put in place
By unknown,
Other hands.

She sang "O Promise Me"
At her sister's wedding,
Giving a gift
That everyone could hear
For a while.

She sang in choir.
Rehearsals were a way
She got away
To sing for more than sixty years.

Other members of the choir
Enjoyed her faithfulness
And they became another family,
A link to a caring community,
To which she gave
All that she had,
And more.

They loved her
Exactly as she was.

They made her feel at home
At last.

She quit the choir,
Suddenly,
Afraid of being ridiculed
For having a failing voice.

I sat
And stood beside her,
Unaware
Of any changes in her ability
To sing,
And keep on singing
On pitch
And strong.

Her eyesight failed.
She withdrew gradually,
Unable to see to sing.
But able to reach into her memory
For notes
And rhythms
Stored for later use.

She died quietly,
Carried away by the music of falling waters
In never ending streams.

The choir sang at her funeral
And now is singing
New songs
She never got to sing.

She is at home
Again,
In music without beginning
Or end.

She gets to sing with Mozart
Every day!

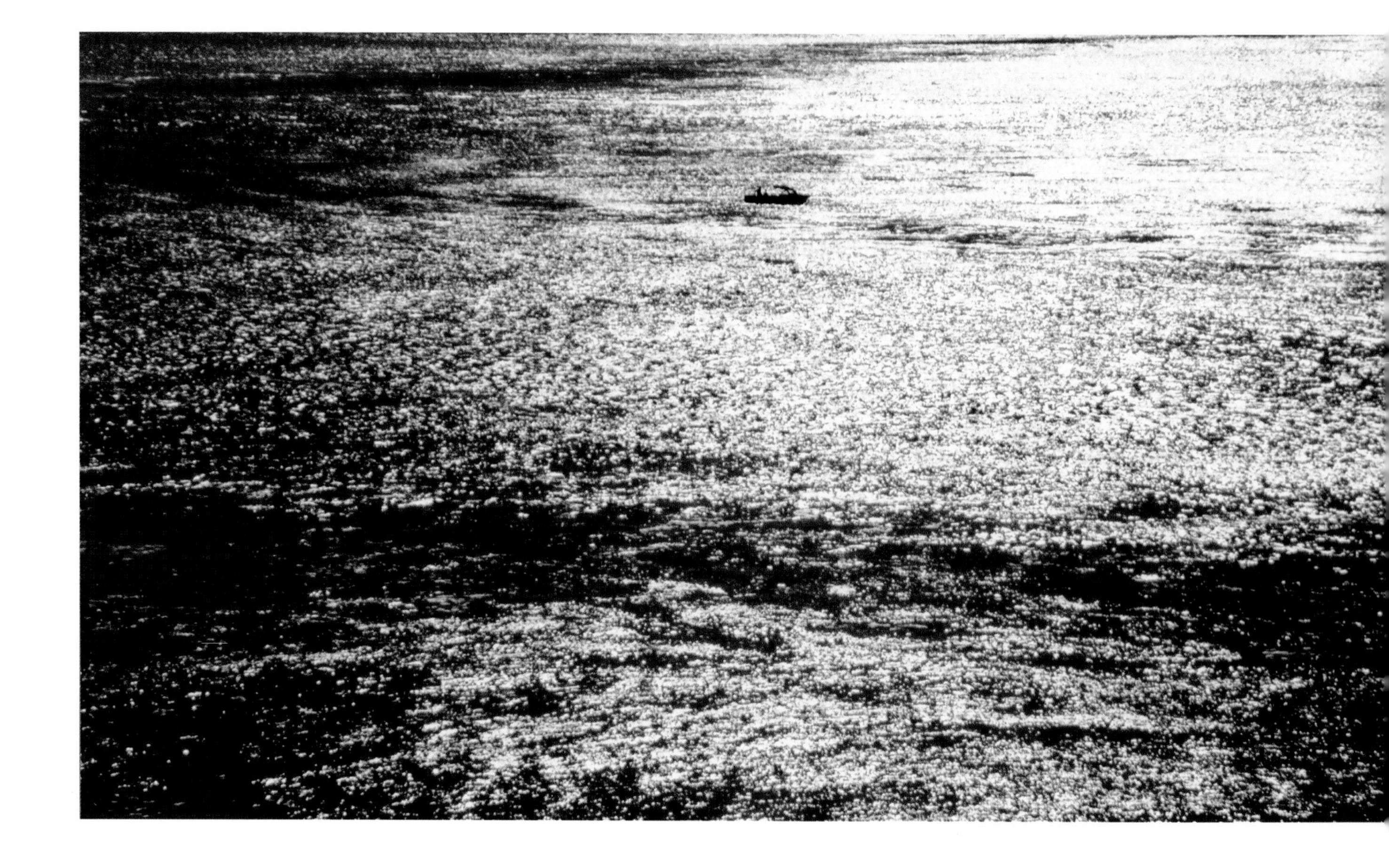

I beat my way
Against the current,
That great stream
Surging through the sea.

06/22/82 | *Between Victoria and Vancouver,* British Columbia 1995

The river almost disappears
In mist
And mystery.

Sunlight would spoil everything!
Sometimes sunshine is too much!

There is a mood,
A sense of brooding
When the air itself is heavy,
Calm,
And solemn.

How deep the river is,
Its thin skin surface gives no clues.

Where the river is going
Lies hidden beyond the nearly
closing of the trees.

I feel like that
Today.
Too much insight,
Too much light,
Would blind me
To the trust I need
To go where some deep,
Internal urgings
Push and pull me,
Meta ta physika.

It is a gift
To sit beside the dying,
Unable to do
Some thing
Except to be,
There.

It is enough
To be present
And aware
That being there,
In weakness,
Is strength.

It is an end
To fear,
And joy,
And all the cares
That trap us
Every day.

It is a time
To do remembering,
When images emerge,
Unbidden,
From the half hidden
Regrets
That moments were wasted,
That opportunities were lost,
That time itself
Does not forgive.

It is a way,
The only way,
To say "Goodbye,"
"God be with you,"
With words,
Within silence.

Jays,
Once companions in the snow,
Are scattered now.
Where?

Partridge erupt,
From the same tree,
Day after day.

We still see
And hear the call
Of occasional crows.

Juncos are lively companions now,
Picking over snow soaked seeds,
Warming themselves
With jittery chatter.

Hawks watch,
Floating,
Silently.

Eagles have returned,
Again,
Screaming at each other.

Is there a connection?

04/08/97

Flight, North of Walker, Minnesota 1998

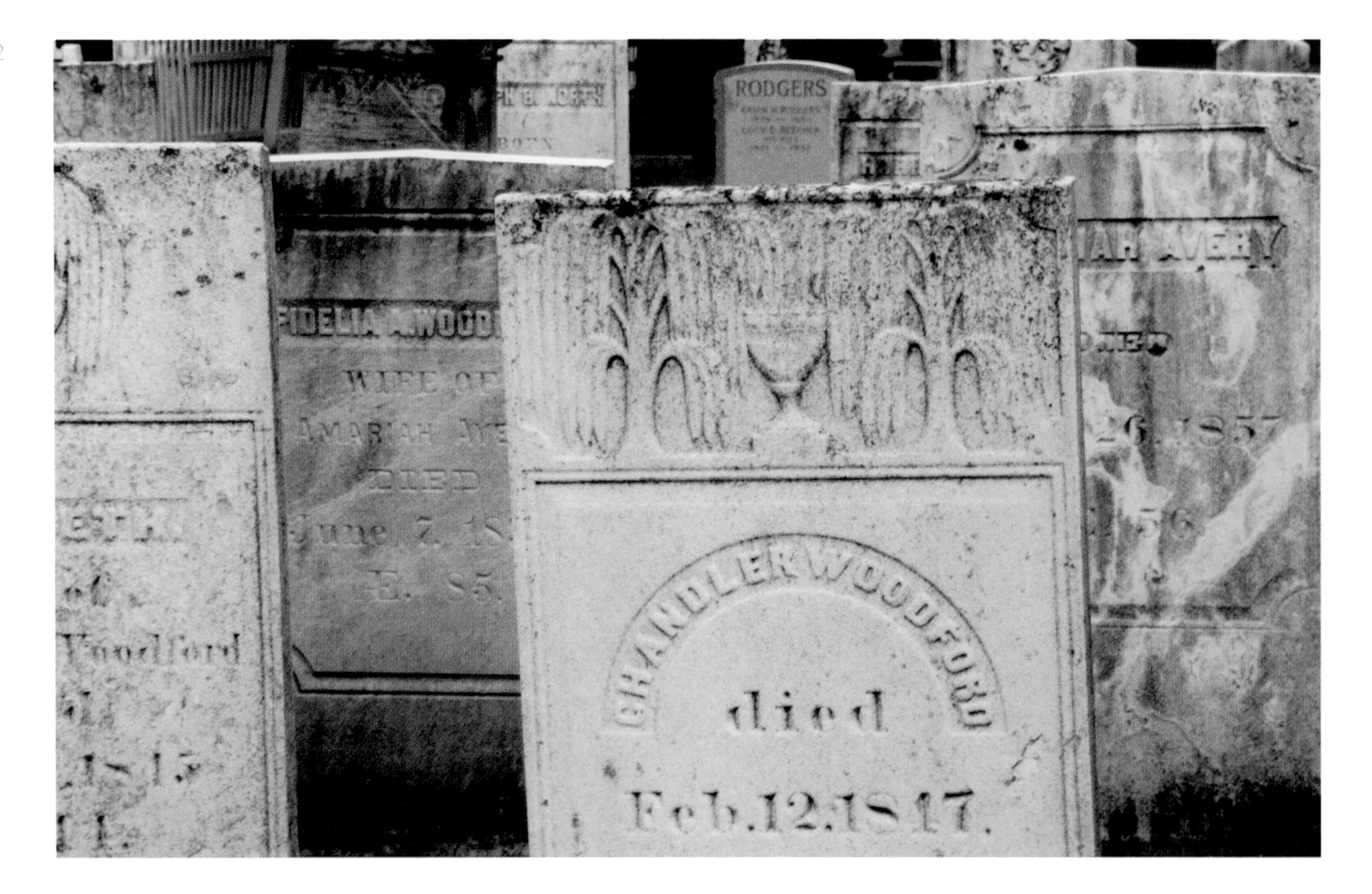

Continuity, Near Simsbury, Connecticut 1998 | 11/19/96

For the first time
My mother,
Who was alive
When you were born,
Is not here
To be aware
That you were born
Again,
Today,
For the first time.

For the first time
You are together again
Away from the cold and snow
That surrounded you
When you were born
For the first time.

For the first time
Your families are complete:
Sisters,
Brothers,
Brothers and sisters,
In one great,
Small space,
Together,
For the first time.

For the first time,
With each other,
You can see
Beyond bickering
And evasive words
Into the great brimming bowl
Of knowing
And forgetting,
For the first time.

For the first time,
All you are
And ever were,
Together,
Is finished,
Finally,
For the first time.

For the first time
Your temporary heartbeats
Echo endlessly,
Silently,
Together,
Around the curved
And empty edges
Of the universe,
For the first time.

For the first time
I am alone,
Here,
In my own way,
For the first time.

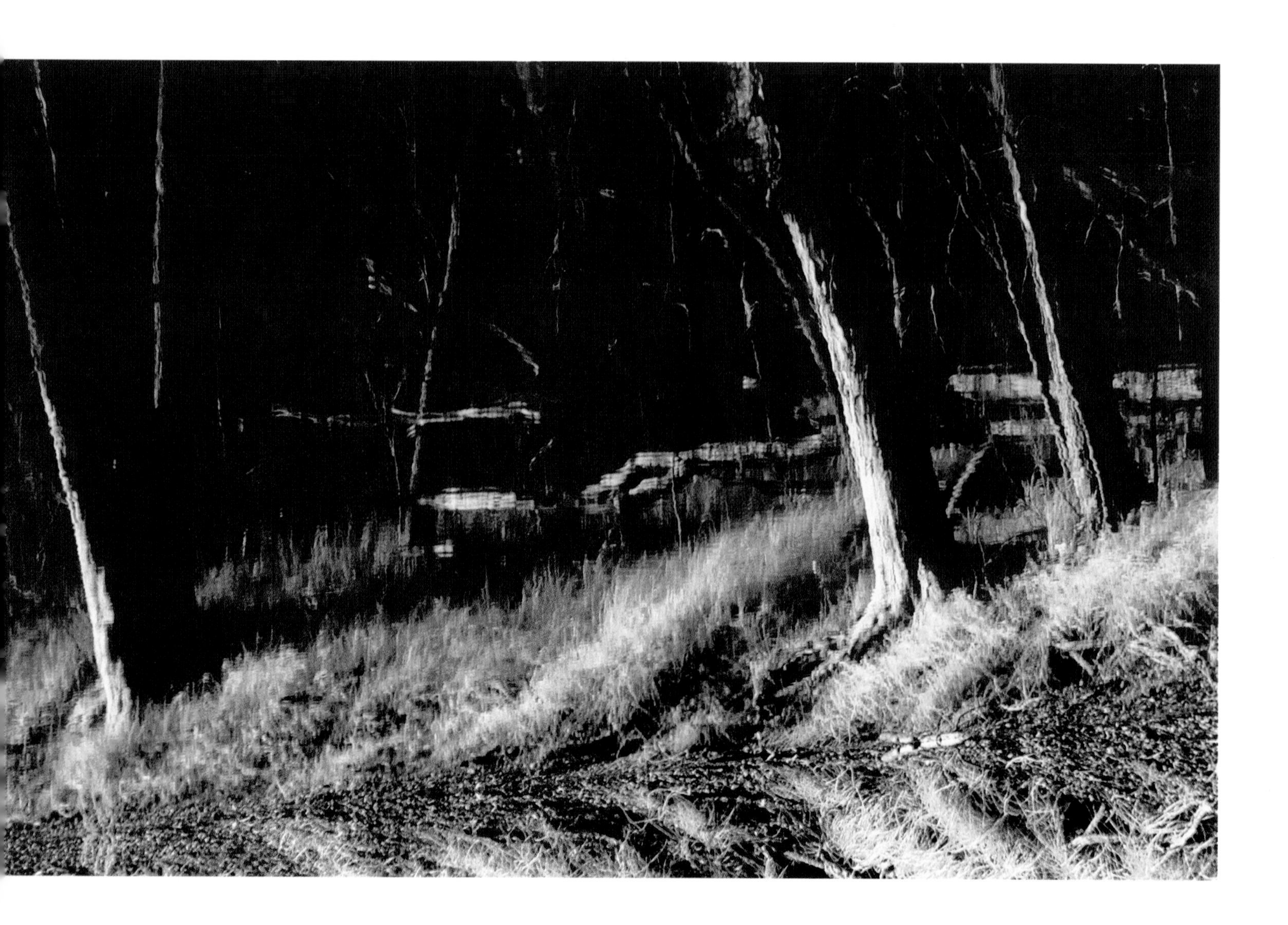

Trees Reflected, Mississippi River, Crow Wing County, Minnesota 2001 (image inverted) | 03/03/00

Because of the light . . .

Because of the light, shadows detail the scale of rocks
and outwash plains end watercourses, abruptly.

greying snows glow in the woods,
recharging the roots of trees
impatient for the greening of Spring.

birches and aspens merge indifferently at
the edges of a long dead lake.

no line defines the sky
shading into ground cloud.

irrelevant dust creates spotlights out
of cloud holes.

distant rain breaks sunlight into
curves of color.

invisible changes merge into
tangible form.

differences become distinctive figures on
a common ground.

the seen and heard congeal from
time to time.

decay creates new realities out of
old possibilities.

impulsive breezes break the flat
slab of the lake into small, immediate mirrors.

bursts of energy erupt with orderly
spontaneity.

transparent glass twists images into
accurate distortions of reality.

we see we cannot see through
surficial skin to what is.

my eyes are seduced
in searching for simplicity.

Because of the light, it is possible to live and hope
until the coming of the night.

From time to time,
On bright blue days,
I see green leaves,
Glossy with fragments of light,
Like wavelets,
Windblown,
Breaking into sharp shards,
Pinpoints of empty whiteness.

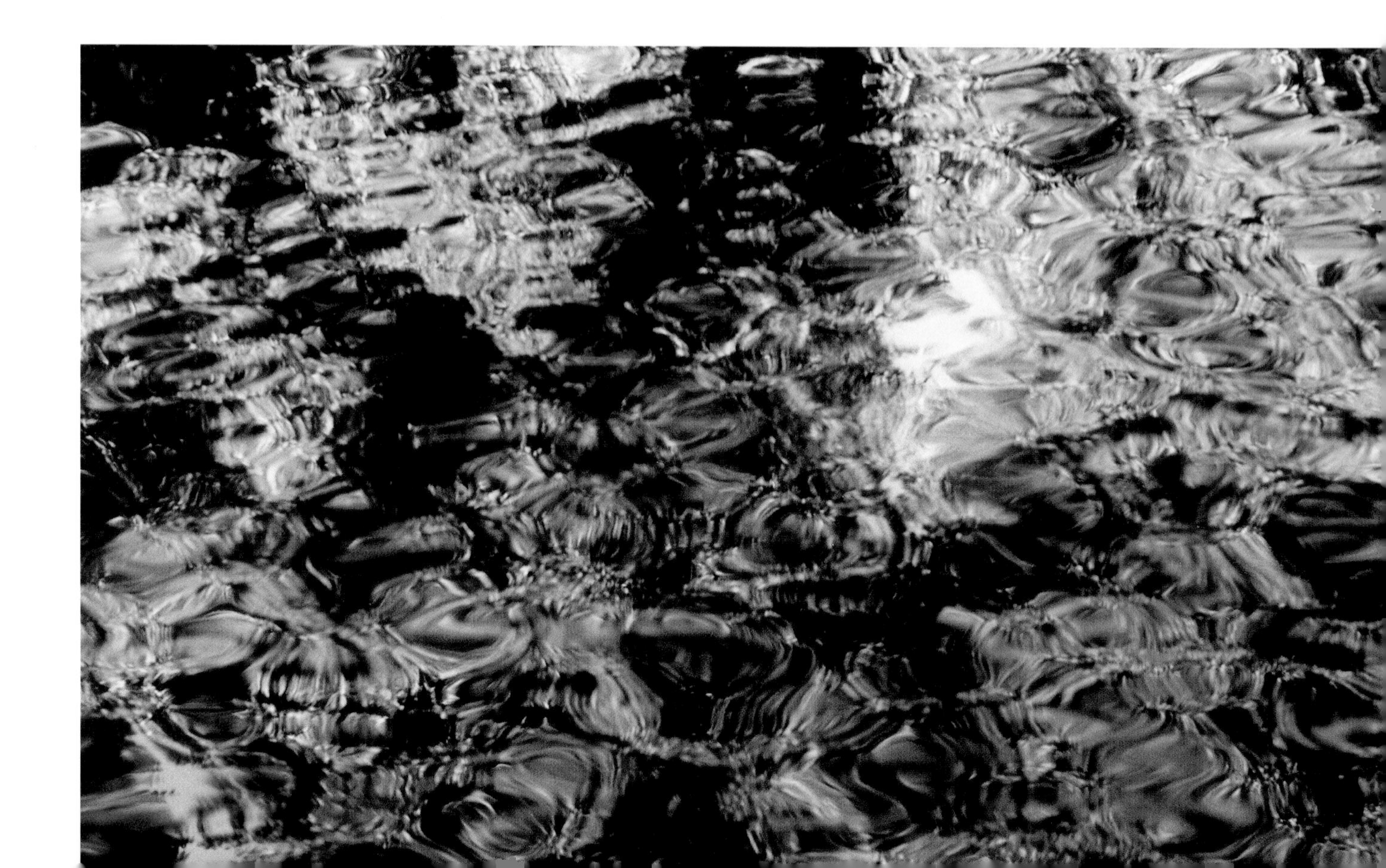

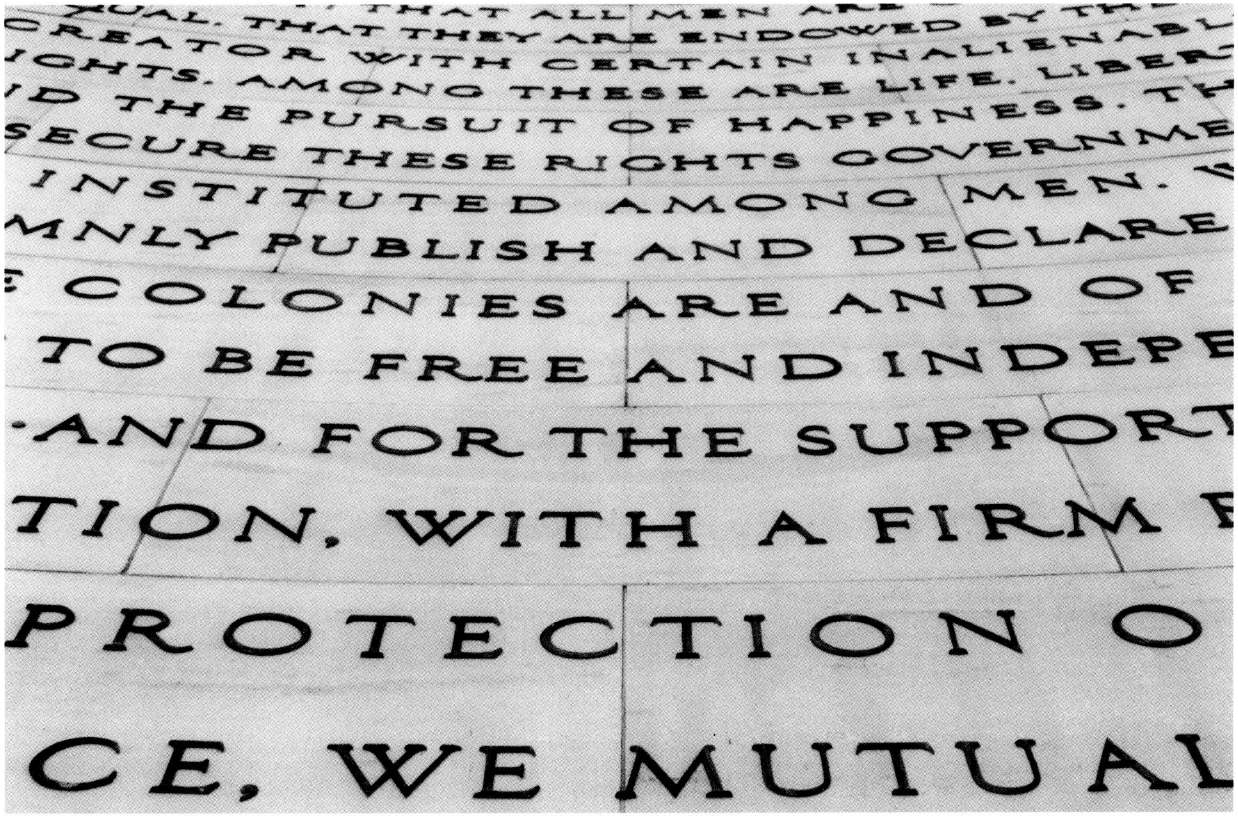

Words work!
How?
By making memory and images,
With no assurance that what I see
Is what you see
With me.

Words may be
Like billiard balls,
Bouncing into each other,
Also caroming around,
Butting into the edges we build
To form a framework
Creating continuity
And stability,
A new reality.

Declaration of Independence, Jefferson Memorial, Washington D.C. 2000 | 10/26/99

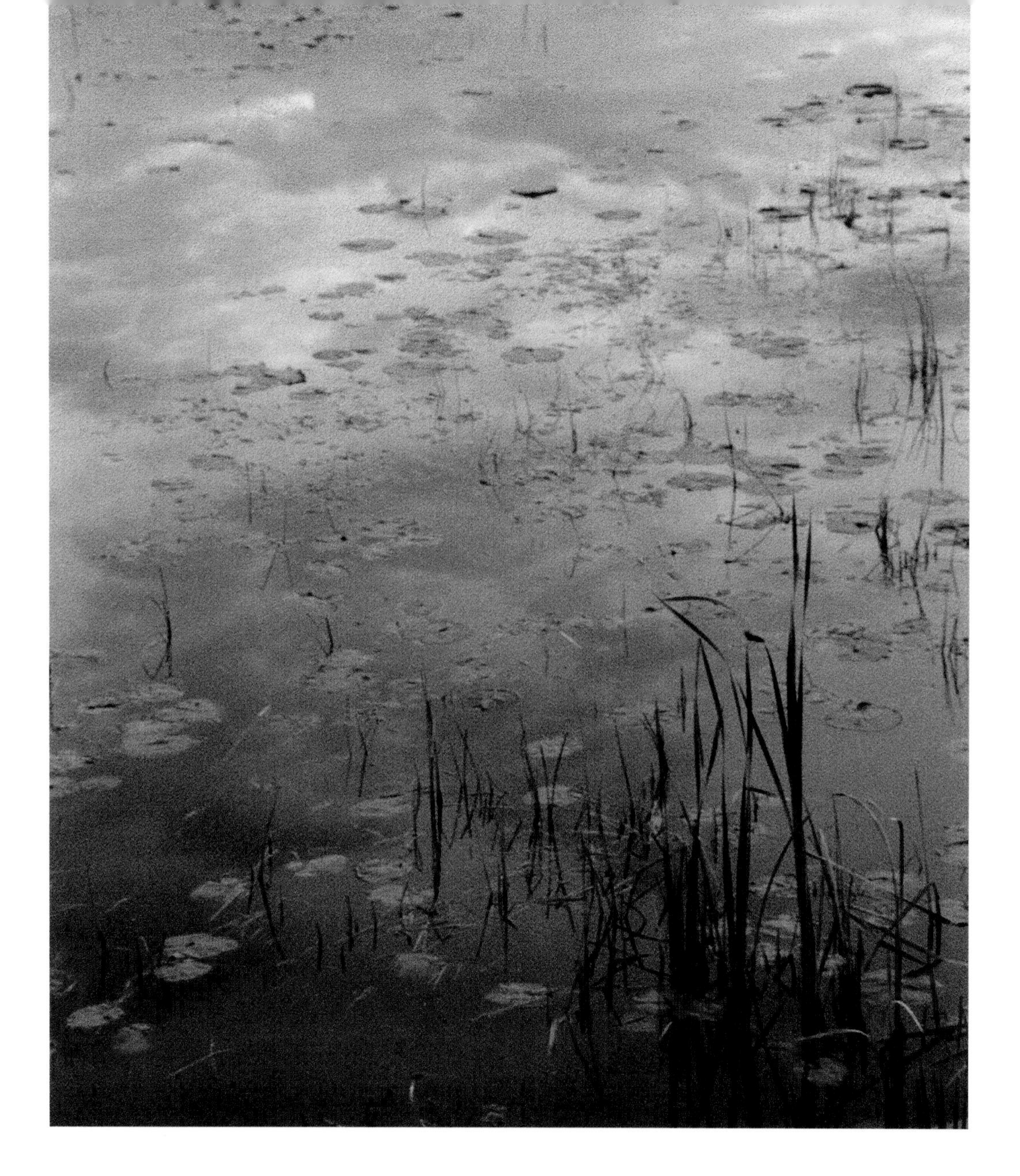

Why go to Giverny?
Monet's water lilies
Are alive!
In Minnesota!

Impressionists taught us to see
What in fact
Is already there.

Where?

On the pellicle of water plants,
On the thin skin of the lake itself,
Reflecting the husks and hulls of
trees themselves,
Their limbs and leaves
Immediately,
So close,
And yet,
So far away!

Transition, Stream, Nisswa, Minnesota 2000 | 10/30/01

Turn out the light.
Turn around with me.
Come to the window.

Do you see,
Above the black
And shredded trees,
How the moon is moving up
Across the frozen lake,
Making moving shadows
In the wrinkled snow?

Stand with me
For a while.

Hold me
For a while.

Look with me
For a while.

Absorb the peace,
The stillness
Holding back the dark
Between tiny diamonds
Flashing in the snow
And sparking in the sky.

Turn out the light.
Stay here with me
A little while,
Longer.

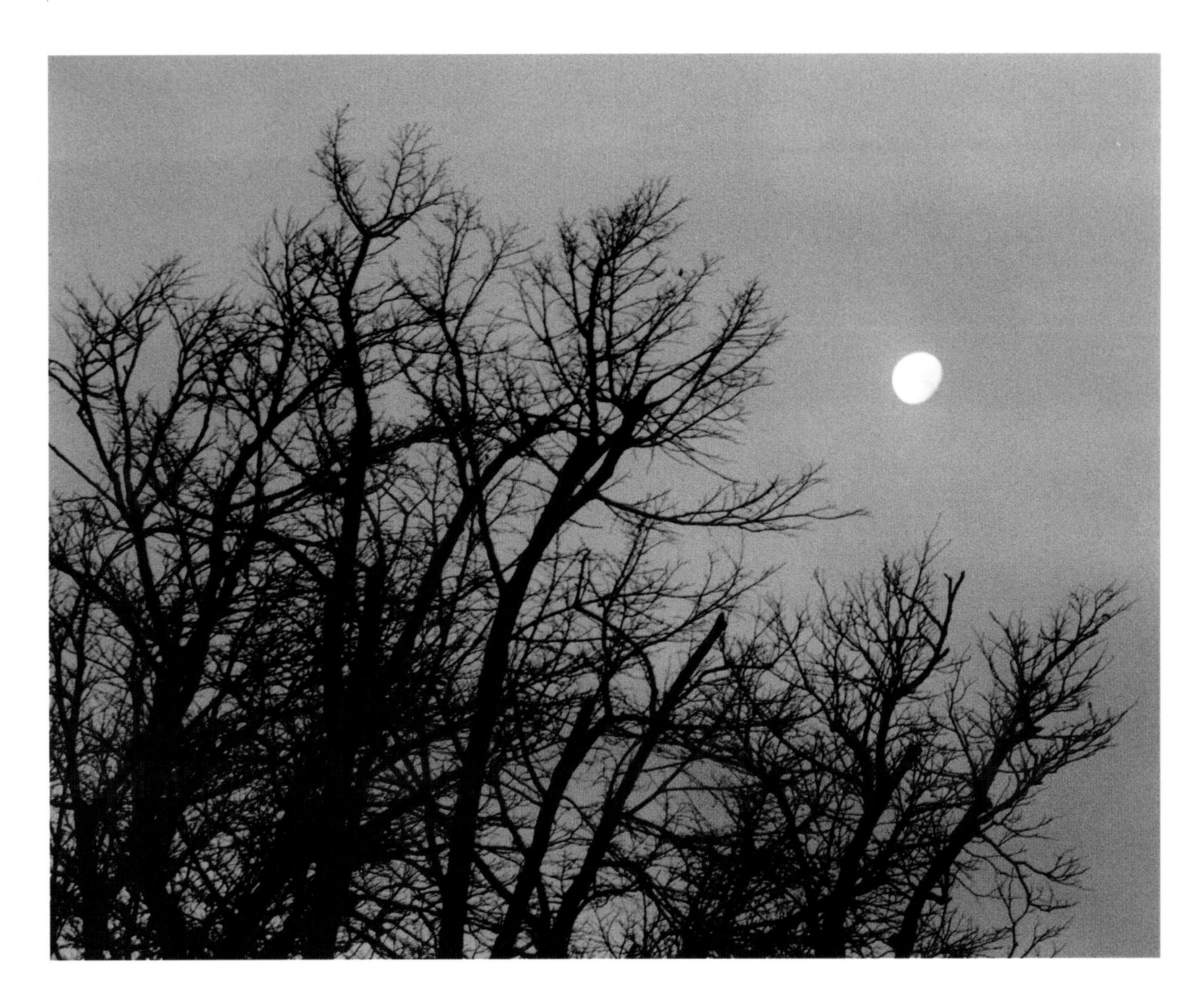

Artist's Statement

The world is there, in a poem.

It is seen there, in words wondrously few and mysteriously powerful, where time stops and eternity is present. We are drawn in and not released, all in the word.

At its best, a photograph is visual poetry, a perceptive expression of thought, emotion, relation, place, a window to an unconsidered moment of light. An image's borders are not real: A telling photograph creates an opening into another dimension which, like the poem, leaves us breathless in time and in space.

Roger Cooper's poetry sang without giving voice for most of his life. His word was unknown to all, including to those images gathering in time for their meeting in verse, here. We have joined these parallel universes, unspoken word and unseen light, better to consider this place and this time that is now and that is ours, but which is neither.

john erickson

Artist's Statement

How do we encounter the world? How does the world present itself to us? The eye, the ear, the nose, taste buds, fingertips all provide us with essential sensory input. But what happens next?

The mind does some matching and mixing, creating new combinations of percepts, concepts. Ideas emerge as intuitions, insights into the "never before." Something meaningful for an instant or for a lifetime is suddenly there, and we are aware. A cluster of internal operations, mostly automatic, sift and sort, pile up perceptions, pigeonhole them or create new categories for apprehending them.

Voila! Something meaningful has taken place, something that breaks into individual reality but also transcends that reality. A kind of "community" is created, often without an intention to do so.

It makes no difference what the originating stimulus is: A poem or a photograph, or some fortuitous combination of them. What makes a difference is the impact they make, severally and together, synergistically or at variance. The impact of poetry and photography is determined in large part by the attention paid by the photographer to the interplay of light and shadow, by the poet's choice and rejection of words and the interstices among them.

Creating a poem is much like a sculptor's work in uncovering the statue hidden in a block of marble. It is there, already, in a mass of experience congealed in words, waiting to be brought to light. A good poem catches our attention and reorganizes our experiencing of the world.

roger cooper

ACKNOWLEDGEMENTS

We wish to express our special appreciation to Chip Borkenhagen, one of the principals of our publisher, EVERGREEN PRESS, for his insight in bringing our art together, for his personal encouragement and for his own remarkable vision, benefitting us and others; to Jean Borkenhagen, also an EVERGREEN PRESS principal, for her warm support and constructive criticism; and to Dr. Robert Steven Bianchi, for the uncommon presence he has been among us.

We are thankful for the skills and creativity of the staff of EVERGREEN PRESS, in particular Mandi Selisker, Bryan Petersen and Jodi Schwen, each of whom has provided unique, truly artistic contributions to whatever beneficial effect IMPRESSIONS may have.

What we hope will touch the reader's soul in IMPRESSIONS is an accumulation of the many positive influences and effects we have been the grateful beneficiaries of through the years given to us. What shortcomings are to be found here are ours, alone.

john erickson and roger cooper